the GIGANTIC book of RUNNING Quotations

the GIGANTIC *book of* RUNNING *Quotations*

Edited and Introduced by **HAL HIGDON**
Foreword by **AMBY BURFOOT**

Skyhorse Publishing

Skyhorse Publishing books may be purchased in bulk at special discounts for sales promotion, corporate gifts, fund-raising, or educational purposes. Special editions can also be created to specifications. For details, contact the Special Sales Department, Skyhorse Publishing, 307 West 36th Street, 11th Floor, New York, NY 10018 or info@skyhorsepublishing.com.

Skyhorse® and Skyhorse Publishing® are registered trademarks of Skyhorse Publishing, Inc.®, a Delaware corporation.

Visit our website at www.skyhorsepublishing.com.

Library of Congress Cataloging-in-Publication Data is available on file.

10 9 8 7 6 5 4 3 2 1

Cover design by David Ter-Avanesyan
Cover photos credit: Getty Images
Interior images: Getty Images

ISBN: 978-1-5107-6629-7
ebook ISBN: 978-1-62636-700-5

Printed in the United States of America

CONTENTS

FOREWORD

I've long believed that many runners have the wrong idea about what it takes to succeed in the mile, the 10K, cross-country, the marathon, or whatever your chosen distance might be. You don't need long legs. You don't need a skinny frame. You don't need a special diet or a secret training plan. You don't even need an over-sized heart capable of pumping vast quantities of oxygen-rich blood to all parts of your body. (Though that's a good thing, no doubt about it.)

What you need is motivation, and lots of it. Enough motivation to stick to a consistent running program. Because without consistency, none of the above (not even a big heart) will improve your performances.

The best motivation comes from a steadfast friend (or many such friends). A literal friend and training partner is a great asset, but not always available. A second option and a constant, always-there-when-you-need-him/her friend is the inspirational running quote. Too stressed by work deadlines to fit in your run? Reach for a great quote. Too fatigued by family responsibilities? A little quote will do you. Too sleepy to get out of bed for your morning run? Make sure you've got a favorite quote close at hand.

I know few lifelong runners who don't have dozens of favorite running quotes—from the Bible, from Shakespeare, from other poets, from songs, from famous leaders, from philosophers, and from many other sources. We post these quotes in all our most important life spaces—at home, at work, in training logs, on calendars, and of course on the refrigerator, where they often battle for space with prized photos of families and friends. We feel lost and somewhat vulnerable if we look around and don't spot one of our revered quotes. We recognized their power; we want to keep them close to us.

I readily recall the key moments of my own evolution as a quote fan. When

I was young, like all children, I had a favorite book that I begged my parents to read over and over again. It was *The Little Engine That Could*, the story of the tiny locomotive that achieved what bigger rivals couldn't simply by repeating "I think I can, I think I can" over and over again. Many decades later, I'm somewhat embarrassed to admit how much this simplistic tale meant to me. Somewhat. But not totally. In fact, I expect *The Little Engine* had more influence on my life than I've ever fully realized.

In junior high, I read dozens of books in the "Chip Hilton" sports series, and there I first encountered the old chestnut, "When the going gets tough, the tough get going." Again, it's ridiculously simple. But also a bit catchy. And I've probably used this quote more often than any other when I needed a burst of extra energy in a tough race or workout.

The older I got, the more great quotes I encountered, and the more diverse. Some from great thinkers, some from fast and famous runners, and some from writers who had a delightfully skewed perspective on life. In my lexicon, the quote both humorous and motivational is a special treasure. I particularly enjoy a number of Lewis Carroll quotes. When I'm on a treadmill, I always think about this observation from the Red Queen: "It takes all the running you can do to keep in the same place. If you want to get somewhere else, you must run at least twice as fast." Now, I know that doesn't sound encouraging, but it always brings a smile to my face, and the smile helps me run smoother.

When daunted by a difficult task, I like to remember one of Alice's conversations from *Alice in Wonderland*. Alice protests the futility of trying to believe in the impossible. But the Queen retorts that Alice obviously hasn't tried very hard, noting, "Why, sometimes I've believed as many as six impossible things before breakfast." Personally, at that early an hour, I'm usually willing to settle for just one or two.

I'll mention just two more favorite quotes. As a runner who has spent forty years striving to stay both fit and competitive, I've always been drawn to the words of 1989 New York City Marathon champion Juma Ikangaa. Ikangaa, a

Tanzanian who raced frequently in the United States, once said: "The will to win means nothing without the will to prepare." This quote will get me out of bed almost any morning, no matter now dark and dreary.

Finally, here's my favorite running quote among all the thousands that you'll find on the pages that follow. It comes from the writings of Dr. George Sheehan, longtime *Runner's World* contributor, who probably coined more memorable and inspirational running phrases than any other author. Anytime you need a boost, Sheehan is sure to provide. The quote: "There are as many reasons for running as there are days in the year, years in my life. I run because I am an animal and a child, an artist and a saint."

I treasure this quote because I believe, as Wordsworth did, that we all contain multitudes. And that we are capable of finding many reasons for our runs—competitive reasons, health reasons, creative reasons, psychological reasons, spiritual reasons. Indeed, we run one day for one purpose, and another day with a completely different goal.

And for each of those goals, we can find a different quote to get us going. Enjoy them all. And treasure every run.

Amby Burfoot
January 2008

INTRODUCTION

In *Through the Looking Glass*, Lewis Carroll puts these words in the Red Queen's mouth: "Now, here, you see, it takes all the running you can do to keep in the same place. If you want to get somewhere else, you must run at least twice as fast as that."

Carroll's classic sequel to *Alice in Wonderland* was published in 1871, a full century before Jim Fixx's *The Complete Book of Running* sold a million copies in hardback and helped launch the running boom. But Carroll was hardly the first writer to tie a phrase to running. "Now bid me run," wrote William Shakespeare, "and I will strive with things impossible." The bard of Avon gave that line to Julius Caeser, though no evidence exists that Caeser ever ran a marathon. Come to think of it, the tale of Pheidippides running from the plains of Marathon into Athens, the legend we base our sport upon, owes more to fiction than to fact.

You will encounter the words of Carroll and Shakespeare in this seminal volume of *Running Wisdom*, compiled from many sources, but you also can enjoy the words of Burfoot, Henderson, Sheehan and Fixx. And a few quotes from Higdon too. As running has matured from boom to a defining movement that has shaped lives, new writers have emerged to stand on the slender shoulders of Amby, Joe, George, Jim and I. Kenny Moore, Tom Derderian and Roger Robinson for example. Olympic champions Emil Zatopek, Frank Shorter and Joan Benoit Samuelson have proved quotable. Their chosen words help enrich the pages of this book of running wisdom.

Lewis Carroll and William Shakespeare to the contrary, it seems that the recording of running bon mots began to thrive in the 1960s, a decade both dark with despair and bright with hope, an era when the Boston Marathon attracted only a few hundred starters, most of them capable of breaking 3 hours. I cashed my first paychecks as a magazine editor, then morphed into a freelance writer, embracing the freeness of that discipline partly because it gave me time to run in daylight. During my early career, I wrote about anything other than long distance running, because who wanted to read about that sport back in 1959?

That was the year I ran my first Boston. We were a scurvy lot, the 150 of us who showed up in Hopkinton, our deeds largely unheralded. And certainly there was little advice offered to those who wanted to conquer the marathon.

That soon would change. In 1966, a high school runner from Kansas named Bob Anderson started what was little more than a newsletter, called *Distance Running News*. It grew in circulation, so three years later Anderson dropped out of college and moved to California, hiring a young staffer from *Track & Field News* named Joe Henderson as editor. They changed the publication's name to *Runner's World* in time for the January 1970 issue, the first issue of the decade when running finally captured the interest of a public that previously assumed running to be a sport confined to the young and restless.

Many who would shape the world of running as we view it today came together about that time. Hopkinton Green, starting point for the Boston Marathon, offered the common meeting ground. Dr. Kenneth Cooper, author of *Aerobics*, ran there in the early 1960s. So did Erich Segal, author of *Love Story*. Henderson first ran Boston in 1967. In 1968, Amby Burfoot, who one day would become editor of *Runner's World*, won the Boston Marathon. That same year and at the Olympic Games in Mexico City, I introduced Joe Henderson to a doctor friend and Boston fellow traveler: George Sheehan. Recruited by Joe, George would go on to become *Runner's World's* most popular columnist as well as a best-selling author. In 1971, I wrote a book titled *On The Run From Dogs and People*, its title borrowed from an article previously published by *Sports Illustrated*. Somewhat of a cult classic, that book remains in print today and provides at least one quote for this book.

All those named above contributed to the growth of a sport that eventually would be accepted by the masses, both those running marathons and watching them. Frank Shorter won the Olympic Marathon in 1972 and after that came Jim Fixx, and in the five decades following a host of running writers quoted in the pages following. They provide us with words of running wisdom.

Use these words as your inspiration and you will be able, as suggested by William Shakespeare, to strive with things impossible. You might even run fast enough to please Lewis Carroll.

—Hal Higdon
Contributing Editor:
Runner's World

CHAPTER ONE

Ready to run?

Starting Line

The most important task for the beginning runner is that you "begin." A simple verb, full of sound and fury, signifying much, to paraphrase Shakespeare. Beginning is a chore most difficult to achieve. Unless you take that first step as a beginner, you are not going anywhere.

But so many individuals have put that first foot forward, taking a first step, even if it is not a running step. They follow with a second step, and this opens a world of hope. Soon a short stroll becomes a longer walk. A short jog becomes a longer run. Then one day you look up and find yourself on the starting line of a marathon surrounded by tens of thousands of individuals who, like you, might have taken their first running steps only months before.

Running comes with a price. Between that first step as a walker or a runner and steps taken during the 26 miles 385 yards of a marathon come moments of pleasure and—let's be honest—moments of pain.

But that goes with the joy of being a runner. And you cannot become a runner unless you first begin. A simple verb, full of sound and fury, leading to a lifetime commitment.

The world is divided into two kinds of people: runners and non-runners.
—Marc Bloom, *The Runner's Bible*

———◆———

In a world that's quickly becoming so fast-paced that multi-tasking is a way of life, runners have managed to find a way to do something that's good for our heads, bodies, and spirits, and that provides wonderful social interaction.
—John Bingham

———◆———

If walking upright first set early human ancestors apart from their ape cousins, it may have been their eventual ability to run long distances with a springing step over the African savanna that influenced the transition to today's human body form. . .
—John Noble Wilford, "Running Extra Miles Sets the Human Apart," *The New York Times,* November 18, 2004

———◆———

Laziness is nothing more than the habit of resting before you get tired.
—Jules Renard

Number one is just to gain a passion for running. To love the morning, to love the trail, to love the pace on the track. And if some kid gets really good at it, that's cool too.

—Pat Tyson

Running removes us briefly from the fragmentation and depersonalization of the digital world.

—Amby Burfoot, *The Runner's Guide to the Meaning of Life*

I can't remember what I was doing before running. I guess shopping, sewing, watching TV—gaining nothing.

—Miki Gorman

I'm afraid the reason so many new runners quit is because they never get past the point of feeling like they have to run.

—John Bingham, "Who Needs a Reason?" *Runners World*

All runners, at one time or another, are beginners.

—*The New York Road Runners Club Complete Book of Running*

It is not so much that I began to run, but that I continued.
  —Hal Higdon

———◆———

Now bid me run,
And I will strive with things impossible,
Yea, get the better of them.
  —Shakespeare, *Julius Caesar*

———◆———

A runner is real when she takes the first step.
  —Clarissa Pinkola Estés, Ph.D.

———◆———

Running is a great investment. Your principal is low. Your rate of return is enormous, and it keeps growing every year. And there are no hidden charges, unless you count an occasional blister.
  —Florence Griffith Joyner and Jon Hanc, *Running for Dummies*

———◆———

Running is elementary. It is elegant in its simplicity.
  —John Bingham, *The Courage to Start*

Just as you write down other important appointments, you need to literally pencil in time for your run. The process itself is empowering. In the few seconds it takes to scribble "run" into a time slot, you make running a part of your life.
    —Jeff Galloway

I'm not saying running could solve all of the world's problems, but I think it would be a good start.
    —John Bingham

If you feel great the first day, like a million dollars, you're an exception.
    —Marc Bloom

If you want to become the best runner you can be, start now. Don't spend the rest of your life wondering if you can do it.
    —Priscilla Welch

Endurance? You've only got to get out there and do it. Face up to it: Man was meant to run.
    —Percy Cerutty

Running is not just exercise; it is a lifestyle.
> —John Bingham, *Running for Mortals: A Commonsense Plan for Changing Your Life with Running*

I put it in historical perspective. This is our heritage; our evolutionary gift, dating back to our days as hunters and gatherers.
> —Stu Mittleman

The most important message I stress to beginners is to learn to love the sport. Like other endeavors, if running is not undertaken properly, it can be difficult and discouraging.
> —Cliff Held

A lot of people say they love running because of how they feel afterward. Not me. Well, I love that, too, but it's also so much fun while I'm out there.
> —Dick Beardsley

In the beginning you likely say, "I run." With more confidence, you say, "I am a runner."
> —Gloria Averbuch

[Y]ou were born to run. Maybe not that fast, maybe not that far, maybe not as efficiently as others. But to get up and move, to fire up that entire energy-producing, oxygen-delivering, bone-strengthening process we call running.
  —Florence Griffith Joyner and Jon Hanc, *Running for Dummies*

⬛◆⬛

Now, here, you see, it takes all the running you can do, to keep in the same place. If you want to get somewhere else, you must run at least twice as fast as that.
  —Lewis Carroll, *Through the Looking-Glass*

⬛◆⬛

When people ask me why I run, I tell them, there's not really a reason, it's just the adrenaline when you start, and the feeling when you cross that finish line, and know that you are a winner no matter what place you got.
  —Courtney Parsons

⬛◆⬛

Running is a thing worth doing not because of the future rewards it bestows, but because of how it feeds our bodies and minds and souls in the present.
  —Kevin Nelson, *The Runner's Book of Daily Inspiration*

For me, running is a lifestyle and an art. I'm more interested in the magic of it than the mechanics.
—Lorraine Moller, four-time New Zealand Olympian

Running is real and relatively simple—but it ain't easy.
—Mark Will-Weber

Every time I walk out the door, I know why I'm going where I'm going and I'm already focused on that special place where I find my peace and solitude.
—Sasha Azevedo

The advice I have for beginners is the same philosophy that I have for runners of all levels of experience and ability—consistency, a sane approach, moderation and making your running an enjoyable, rather than dreaded, part of your life.
—*Bill Rodgers' Lifetime Running Plan*

Starting is scary. It is for everyone. . . . I never allowed my eyes to meet those of other runners, because I was afraid of seeming like an impostor.
—John Bingham, *The Courage to Start*

Do something that involves use of the body. How can you hope to run when you spend the whole day standing still? How can you hope to master your own body when your body is the slave of a machine?
  —Brian Ganville, "The Olympian"

If someone could find a way to bottle motivation, he would make a fortune.
  —Hal Higdon

It's very hard in the beginning to understand that the whole idea is not to beat the other runners. Eventually you learn that the competition is against the little voice inside you that wants to quit.
  —George Sheehan

When I first started running, I was so embarrassed I'd walk when cars passed me. I'd pretend I was looking at the flowers.
  —Joan Benoit Samuelson

Running is the classical road to self-consciousness, self-awareness, and self-reliance.
  —Noel Carroll

My first understanding was that you could not become a distance runner quickly. I began gradually, not doing too much.
—Henry Rono

———————

I believe in gradual experimentation with running shoes.
—Bill Rodgers

———————

Running is the most elemental sport there is. We are genetically programmed to do it. One might even say we are the free-ranging, curious, restless creatures that we are because of running.
—John Jerome, *The Elements of Effort*

———————

Not just exercise, but a way to get in touch with and reclaim myself in an often fragmenting world, running also serves as a powerful antidote to clinical depression, a metaphor for the creative process, and, in its most profound moments, a spiritual practice.
—Alison Townsend

———————

What I tell women is that anybody can become a runner if she really wants to.
—Priscilla Welch

I was running since I was ten. Since grade one at school, people looked at me and thought, oh gosh, she can really run, she's a natural.
　　—Cathy Freeman

—◆—

Running is like going to a spring: Each of us drinks our fill, and new runners come, pushing aside those in front.
　　—Michael Sandrock

—◆—

Running is the kind of sport where, once it becomes part of your daily routine, there's very little attrition. That's what sets the running boom apart from other booms.
　　—Frank Shorter

—◆—

Too many people have refused to begin running or have quickly dropped out of running programs because they "have no talent for it." Ridiculous. Talent has nothing to do with it. The only thing that matters is mental discipline.
　　—Amby Burfoot, *The Principles of Running*

No one will burn out doing aerobic running. It is too much anaerobic running, which the American scholastic athletic system tends to put young athletes through, that burns them out.
—Arthur Lydiard

On my first day as a runner, I owned nine motorcycles, two cars, a camper, a garden tractor, a riding lawn mower, and a gas-powered weed whacker. I was never in danger of having to exert myself.
—John Bingham, *The Courage to Start*

To change into my baggy shorts and faded Berkeley tank top with the rainbow across the chest, pull my purple running shoes on, and just go, out the door and away, my body emptied of anything but movement through air and what that movement makes of me.
—Alison Townsend

I found myself starting over and needed an outlet, a way to channel the seething debris of rage left over from the divorce and my slowly deteriorating self-esteem and confidence. Running seemed to fit the bill. That, and a martial arts program.
—Donna Isaacson

I protested that I was weak and not fit to run, but the coach sent me for a physical examination and the doctor said that I was perfectly well. So I had to run, and when I got started I felt I wanted to win. But I only came in second. That was the way it started.

—Emil Zatopek

The creative juices can really start flowing when runners are immersed in the wonderful feeling that accompanies the rhythm of running.

—Florence Griffith Joyner and John Hanc, *Running for Dummies*

My greatest challenge when I first started running was overcoming the stares I would get. I began running in 1967, and no other women were out there. I ran around a track and it was so uncomfortable because the men would make comments and I didn't like how they would look at me. I overcame it by running without my contact lenses and pretending the guys weren't there.

—Renita, runner from Sarasota, Florida

Set a goal and a program for yourself, and everything else will follow. Guaranteed.

—Amby Burfoot, *The Principles of Running*

When you experience the run, you regress back to the mandrill on the savannah eluding the enclosing pride of lions that is planning to take your very existence away.
     —Shawn Found

⟹•⟸

For the novice runner, I'd say to give yourself at least two months of consistently running several times a week at a conversational pace before deciding whether you want to stick with it. Consistency is the most important aspect of training at this point.
     —Frank Shorter

⟹•⟸

We were meant to run, and we do so naturally when left to our own devices.
     —Amby Burfoot, *The Runner's Guide to the Meaning of Life*

⟹•⟸

Physical fitness is not only one of the most important keys to a healthy body, it is the basis of dynamic and creative intellectual activity.
     —John F. Kennedy

We're talking about a social movement. It was something that . . . was growing, the idea that you could train at any age, that almost anyone could run a marathon if they ran slow enough, and were patient and drank enough liquid along the way.

—Kenny Moore on the birth of the running movement in the 1970s

It did not have a spokesman yet. It was still a private thing, where you snuck off to run in old sweats.

—Kenny Moore

Fitness has to be fun. If it is not play, there will be no fitness. Play, you see, is the process. Fitness is merely the product.

—George Sheehan

[I]n running (like religion), it's the converts who are likely to exhibit the most zeal. And for that reason, the continuing influx of average beginning runners will always be the lifeblood of this sport.

—Mark Will-Weber

I run because I am an animal. I run because it is part of my genetic wiring. I run because millions of years of evolution have left me programmed to run. And, finally, I run because there's no better way to see the sun rise and set.

—Amby Burfoot, *The Runner's Guide to the Meaning of Life*

Everyone who has run knows that its most important value is in removing tension and allowing a release from whatever other cares the day may bring.

—Jimmy Carter

Why should I practice running slow? I already know how to run slow. I want to learn to run fast.

—Emil Zatopek

I always tell beginning runners: Train your brain first. It's much more important than your heart or legs.

—Amby Burfoot, *The Principles of Running*

In short, running can change your entire outlook on life and make a new person out of you.

—Marc Bloom, *The Runner's Bible*

When I got to the starting line, I didn't even know where to stand.
—Grete Waitz, *Run Your First Marathon*

———

Non-runners may not believe how beneficial running can be, but it's true. Running has rocked people's lives—improving the way they look, the way they feel, the way they think, and the way they look at life.
—Florence Griffith Joyner and John Hanc, *Running for Dummies*

———

Look at me: a natural distance runner, wiry and muscular, trained down to gristle. We are the *infantry* of running. Your four-forty and eight-eighty men, these are your cavalry. The sprinters are your shock troops, your commandos.
—John L. Parker, Jr., *Once a Runner*

———

You don't need any skill to run. . . . Every 3-year-old knows how to run.
—Amby Burfoot, *The Runner's Guide to the Meaning of Life*

———

I always cringe inside when people say running comes naturally to me, that training is an uplifting joy. That's not why I race well. I'm competitive.
—Eamonn Coghlan

May your road ahead be a smooth one.
>—Grete Waitz and Gloria Averbuch, *Run Your First Marathon*

The longer the stride the better, but one must never try to take long strides. To overstride oneself is the world of all faults in running, and it is certain to happen if the runner attempts to lengthen his stride.
>—Harry Andrews

I wasn't nervous the first time because I didn't know what to be nervous about. I had no idea what I was in for.
>—Grete Waitz, *Run Your First Marathon*

Running has taught me, perhaps more than anything else, that there's no reason to fear starting lines . . . or other new beginnings.
>—Amby Burfoot, *The Runner's Guide to the Meaning of Life*

If you have ever been around a runner who has just broken a barrier—say suddenly being able to run a 10, 9, 8, or 7-minute mile—then you understand the magic.
>—Jeff Galloway

I could run very fast. After all, in Alabama, all we kids had to do was run, so we ran.

  —Jesse Owens

As the noted saying goes—training is 90 percent physical and 10 percent mental, but look out for that 10 percent.

  —Grete Waitz and Gloria Averbuch, *Run Your First Marathon*

That's the beauty of starting lines: Until you begin a new venture, you never know what awaits you.

  —Amby Burfoot, *The Runner's Guide to the Meaning of Life*

CHAPTER TWO

The running personality

Running to Form

The human body consists of one hundred trillion cells. That is a number so immense that the mind within that body almost cannot comprehend it. But when we lace our shoes, step through the door and move into the environment to engage in the activity we love most, every one of those cells shifts into motion.

They are put in motion by the heart. Not the heart of cardiologists, but the heart of philosophers, who look within the body and even within the mind. "The desire to run comes from deep within us," wrote Dr. Sheehan, "from the unconscious, the instinctive, the intuitive."

I became a runner for admittedly mundane reasons while a sophomore in high school: to win a letter in track and impress my girlfriend of the moment. The letter and the girlfriend have long passed from my life, but running remains a part of that life and always will as long as I have the heart to push those one hundred trillion cells out the door each day.

We are different, in essence, from other men.
　　　—Emil Zatopek

———✦———

Coffee doesn't do it for me; it's running that gets me going.
　　　—Joan Benoit Samuelson

———✦———

I am very determined and the sport is my passion. I believe I am born for running.
　　　—Cathy Freeman

———✦———

Running isn't simply a discipline. It can become like a compulsion—it can become like a god. If you worship this god, you forget everything else. And when you lose this god, you've got nothing.
　　　—Alberto Salazar

———✦———

To run a world record, you have to have the absolute arrogance to think you can run a mile faster than anyone who's ever lived; and then you have to have the absolute humility to actually do it.
　　　—Herb Elliott

It takes a lot more than ability to run fast; it takes the ability to keep coming back and keep coming back.
—Benji Durden

<hr>

I run, therefore I am. And given the years improved fitness adds to our lives, if I did not run, maybe I would no longer be.
—Hal Higdon

<hr>

Even when I'm running I smile because I know that I don't have to.
—John Bingham, "Who Needs a Reason?" *Runners World*

<hr>

"Women have more stamina," she said. "I knew it before liberation."
—Nurse Phillips in Max Apple's "Carbo-Loading"

<hr>

I ran and ran every day, and I acquired a sense of determination, this sense of spirit that I would never, never, give up, no matter what else happened.
—Wilma Rudolph

[Running] pervades my life. I wouldn't go so far as to say it has crept into other parts of my life; I would rather say it has become its own part of my life.
  —Larry Smith

<hr />

I've always got such high expectations for myself. I'm aware of them, but I can't relax them.
  —Mary Decker Slaney

<hr />

The desire to run comes from deep within us—from the unconscious, the instinctive, the intuitive.
  —George Sheehan

<hr />

Why did I get seriously involved in running? I can't put my finger on one specific thing. I became a runner because it suited my personality. It suited me as an individual. There may be a lot of different reasons, but, somehow, they all came together.
  —Bill Rodgers

What am I doing—nobody cares. It's just personal satisfaction.
> —Kenny Moore, American fourth-place finisher in the 1972 Olympic
> Marathon

———⊰•⊱———

Every run is a great run!
> —Sasha Azevedo

———⊰•⊱———

Like so many runners, if I don't run, I don't feel right. I don't feel relaxed; I don't enjoy eating.
> —Fred Lebow

———⊰•⊱———

The key ingredient, in my opinion, to successful mental training is what I refer to as a "warrior attitude."
> —Bob Glover and Shelly-Lynn Florence Glover, *The Competitive*
> *Runner's Handbook*

On those mornings when I was tempted to roll over and fall asleep again, I imagined my racing rivals leaping out of bed and roaring out the front door on a ten-mile workout. The thought so terrified me that I was generally lacing up my shoelaces within five minutes.

  —Amby Burfoot

———◆———

I began running after I became a writer. Since being a writer requires sitting at a desk for hours, I figured that without exercising I'd get out of shape. That was twenty-two years ago.

  —Haruki Murakami

———◆———

The thing I have always liked best about runners is the camaraderie.

  —Kathrine Switzer

———◆———

Running is such a part of my life. If I were never to run another marathon, I would still do two-hour runs.

  —Joan Benoit Samuelson

Eating is not a commitment, it is just something you do. That's what running is to me.

—Larry Smith

<hr />

[R]unning asks that I engage in a practice as difficult, disciplined, and liberating as the writing I do much of the rest of the time.

—Alison Townsend

<hr />

A guy who has run twenty Boston Marathons was once asked, "Don't you feel like skipping a day when it's raining?" The old road warrior replied, "If you start skipping runs because the weather's too lousy, pretty soon you start missing runs because the weather's too nice!"

—Florence Griffith Joyner and John Hanc, *Running for Dummies*

<hr />

Every day, I stop halfway through my run for five minutes, look around, and enjoy the surroundings. I'm reminded of why I do this and why I love it so much.

—Anita Ortiz

[W]hen you actually race [famous runners], you don't want to hear about their being the stuff of legend. You want flesh and blood, preferably flesh covered with a slothful six or seven percent body fat and blood running a little low on hemoglobin. You want to see an arm action start to labor, a back stiffen. You want mortality, not legend.

—Kenny Moore

I didn't enjoy running at first. I thought it was boring. Running in soccer was part of the game so it was okay, but not running for the sake of running.

—Ray Steffen

There is nothing quite so gentle, deep, and irrational as our running—and nothing quite so savage, and so wild.

—Bernd Heinrich, *Why We Run: A Natural History*

Non-runners can add some counterbalance to our fanaticism. Show me a real runner and I will show you someone who has, at least on occasion, become too wrapped up in the sport.

—Mark Will-Weber

I always run alone, away from phones and stress. Running is a major part of my life because it keeps me sane.
  —Michael Roux, Jr., executive chef, Le Gavroche, London

⟹◦⟸

People ask why I run. I say, "If you have to ask, you will never understand." It is something only those select few know. Those who put themselves through pain, but know, deep down, how good it really feels.
  —Erin Leonard

⟹◦⟸

No other sport is as democratic as running.
  —Florence Griffith Joyner and John Hanc, *Running for Dummies*

⟹◦⟸

You talk to enough runners, you'll find out how superstitious many of us are.
  —Dick Beardsley

⟹◦⟸

I think it's good to be able to drive yourself.
  —Priscilla Welch

Years ago, the picture of people running marathons was these lean, mean Type-A male running machines, but today people running are your neighbors, just regular people.

—Tracy Sundlun, Executive Vice President, Elite Racing

Your toughness is made up of equal parts persistence and experience. You don't so much outrun your opponents as outlast and outsmart them, and the toughest opponent of all is the one inside your head.

—Joe Henderson

Coaching an elite runner is something like driving an expensive car. The coach's main job is to steer.

—John Babington

Runners are the Don Quixotes of the world, forever flailing at windmills, sometimes laughed at, rarely understood.

—Michael Sandrock

A miler is the aristocrat of running. A miler is the closest thing to a thorough-bred horse that exists on two legs.
　　—John L. Parker, Jr., *Once a Runner*

———※———

Running is the perfect sport for business travelers. While on location in Los Angeles, I actually bought one of those maps that show the celebrity homes and ran around looking for them.
　　—Jill Cordes

———※———

Running allows me to recharge my batteries. A good run adds a little bounce to my step.
　　—George W. Bush

———※———

[H]e knows no fear and will not listen to the warnings we hopelessly recite: the jarred spine, ruined cartilage, wrecked knees and ankles, fractured shins, the mysterious sudden heart attack in the bloom of life, the neck broken on the expensive beach. . .
　　—Len Otto, "We Cannot Save Him"

A coach can be like an oasis in the desert of a runner's lost enthusiasm.
—Ken Doherty

———

Coaching is an art and I'm not going to let anyone change me.
—Marty Stern

———

As far as being a coach, it's always fascinated me. It's a greater responsibility than most people give it credit for because you're dealing with people.
—Steve Prefontaine

———

I was always a great bundle of energy. As a child, instead of walking, I would run. And so running, which is a pain to a lot of people, was always a pleasure to me because it was so easy.
—Roger Bannister

———

For me, running is a great way to jump-start my day, boost my energy, and have a few minutes to plan and prioritize my schedule.
—Michael Dell

The true competitive runner, simmering in his own existential juices, endured his melancholia the only way he knew how; gently, together with those few others who also endured it, yet very much alone.

    —John L. Parker, Jr., *Once a Runner*

—♦—

I love testing myself more than I fear being beaten, and front running is the ultimate test. You need total, irrevocable commitment to see the race through to the end or it cannot justify your effort.

    —Ron Clarke

—♦—

I like it, the way I live, but I can't explain the satisfaction to people who do not run. . . . Once you know international racing, you can't just ease off a bit. It has to be one or the other, as hard as you can, or just for fun.

    —Grete Waitz

—♦—

It may seem odd to hear a coach say this, but I think a really great training partner is more important than a coach.

    —Joan Nesbit, coach and world-class runner

All my life people have been telling me, 'You're too small, Pre,' 'You're not fast enough, Pre,' 'Give up your foolish dream, Steve.' But they forget something: I have to win.

—Steve Prefontaine

———◆———

I've never known a runner who had as much patience as he needed.

—Amby Burfoot, *The Runner's Guide to the Meaning of Life*

———◆———

It's something in me, deep down, that makes me different in a race.

—Eamonn Coghlan

———◆———

Any kind of athlete, dancer, gymnast, or figure skater is dependent on the body, not on a machine. It's very pure. You can't hide it.

—Michelle Gifford in *New York City Ballet Workout*

———◆———

Running is a way of life for me, just like brushing my teeth. If I don't run for a few days, I feel as if something's been stolen from me.

—John A. Kelley

We're all professionals. Rules don't mean anything.
    —Frank Shorter, testifying before the President's Commission on
       Olympic Sports

———⊰◆⊱———

I was born to run. I love to run. It's almost like the faster I go, the easier it becomes.
    —Mary Decker Slaney

CHAPTER THREE

Tips, advice, and other observations

Going Into Training

What is the difference between running and training? Many runners probably do not even realize that there might be a difference, but one does exist. Running is simply when you run. Training is when you run with a purpose, a goal, a target at the end of the tunnel, be it a 5-K race or a marathon.

We often attach ourselves to both definitions. We run. We train. Some days we cross-train. And some days we rest, which is a form of training in the sense that you occasionally must rest your muscles so that you may run or train or cross-train again. We might do one or the other on any given day, or week, or year, or career.

Perhaps this makes running more complicated that it need be. Fortunately for those who prefer to strain their muscles rather than strain their brains, a wide body of literature exists telling them how to run or train or cross-train and when to rest. Books. Magazine articles. Training programs on the Internet that you can download into your computer or print and post on your refrigerator to guide you on your daily journeys.

All praise those who guide us.

Everyone is an athlete. The only difference is that some of us are in training, and some are not.
  —George Sheehan

———⟫⟐⟪———

Training is principally an act of faith. The athlete must believe in its efficacy: he must believe that through training he will become fitter and stronger.
  —Franz Stampfl

———⟫⟐⟪———

What I did in those early months wasn't "training." It was more about trying not to get hurt than trying to get better.
  —John Bingham, *No Need for Speed: A Beginner's Guide to the Joy of Running*

———⟫⟐⟪———

Running is one of the best solutions to a clear mind.
  —Sasha Azevedo

———⟫⟐⟪———

Training of female athletes is so new that the limits of female possibility are still unknown.
  —Katherine Dunn

What the years have shown me is that running clarifies the thinking process as well as purifies the body. I think best—most broadly and fully—when I am running.
  —Amby Burfoot, *The Runner's Guide to the Meaning of Life*

Two months before the 1952 Olympic Games in Helsinki, the doctors said I must not compete. I had a gland infection in my neck. Well, I didn't listen and what happened? Three golds.
  —Emil Zatopek

Putting miles in your training log is like putting money in the bank. You begin to draw interest on it immediately.
  —Hal Higdon

Injuries made me a cross-training believer.
  —Florence Griffith Joyner

In my opinion, nothing beats a treadmill workout when you don't want to run outside. A good movie, some water, and a little ventilation are all you need.
  —Florence Griffith Joyner

To exercise at or near capacity is the best way I know of reaching a true intro-spective state. If you do it right, it can open all kinds of inner doors.
——Al Oerter

⟭◆⟬

At the highest level, it's interesting to think of what, out of all the training, makes the difference. In Joanie's case, it was running those certain loops very fast.
——Frank Shorter on Joan Benoit Samuelson

⟭◆⟬

As time goes on, I am more into alternative training.
——Grete Waitz

⟭◆⟬

[M]ost of my early training was experimental. I tested theories and techniques on myself. If they worked, I'd pass them on to my friends.
——Ted Corbitt

⟭◆⟬

Of course, I know all the gear in the world won't make me a better runner. Only time and effort do that. But all the gadgets over the years have sure made my training a lot more interesting—and fun.
——John Bingham, "Ready for Takeoff," *Runners World*

First, I figured out the time I thought the mile should be run in. Second, I started testing my theories and particularly my own constitution and capabilities; the result of this study soon convinced me that the then existing records at the distance were by no means good.

—Walter George

We are obviously not far from our limit of safety. If we doubled our speed of movement . . . athletics would become a highly dangerous pastime.

—Archibald Hill in 1927 on the dangers of too much running

The most important day in any running program is rest. Rest days give your muscles time to recover so you can run again. Your muscles build in strength as you rest.

—Hal Higdon

Two- and three-mile events are my objective at the moment. I am out to build up stamina and only racing in those events will help me. It was stamina that beat me when I was away at the Games, and I do not want it to happen again.

—John Landy

By changing the training techniques and attitudes that had previously domi-nated running, [Bill Bowerman, Kenneth Cooper, and Arthur Lydiard] helped make it possible for running to be more than a sport for elite young athletes (nearly all of them male).

 —Joe Henderson, *Running 101*

[Running] transported him, taking his mind to another place, very deep within. Like prayer.

 —Richard Christian Matheson, "Third Wind"

[Scientific testing] can't determine how the mind will tolerate pain in a race. Sometimes, I say, "Today I can die."

 —Gelindo Bordin

The essential thing in life is not so much conquering as fighting well.

 —Baron de Coubertin, founder of the modern Olympic Games

The ability to concentrate is the single element that separates the merely good athlete from the great ones. Concentration is the hallmark of the elite runner.

 —William P. Morgan

Training is like putting money in a bank. You deposit money, and then you can take it out.

  —Fred Lebow

———❖———

It's like a car starting. There's an immense amount of energy you need to start the car, but once you're rolling, it's easy.

  —John Landy on starting training

———❖———

The battles that count aren't the ones for gold medals. The struggles within yourself—the invisible, inevitable battles inside all of us—that's where it's at.

  —Jesse Owens

———❖———

The human body can do so much. Then the heart and spirit must take over.

  —Sohn Kee-Chung, winner of the 1936 Olympic Marathon

———❖———

When running to fill a time quota . . . you can't make that time pass any faster by rushing, so you settle into a pace that feels right to you at the moment. Each minute above a quota is a little victory.

  —Joe Henderson

If you talk to an elite or near-elite American distance runner today, they'll tell you that the primary aim of their training is to avoid injury. If you had talked to a similar athlete 25 years ago—somebody doing the '82 Boston, for example—he would have told you the idea of training was to run fast.
> —Tom Derderian, coach of the Greater Boston Track Club

A lot of people think that they can "sweat out" a fever by running. They think that running will help their immune system fight it off. That's wrong.
> —David Nieman, Ph.D., head of the Human Performance
> Laboratory, Appalachian State University

Dancing and running shake up the chemistry of happiness.
> —Mason Cooley

Everything changed the day I understood that if I was to become a runner, I would have to run with the body I had.
> —John Bingham, *The Courage to Start*

It's as if you set your destination . . . and then you figure out how you're getting there from where you are. So you plan your training and your diet, and figure out what else you need to do to get you from this point to that point.
— Lorraine Moller

⟨⧫⟩

I didn't get a chance to voice my opinion on whether or not I *wanted* to run. I'd joined the Women's Army Corps and when Aunt Sam yelled, "Double-time, march!" that's exactly what we all did—no matter if our feet were blistered and our lungs felt ready to pop.
— Roberta B. Jacobson

⟨⧫⟩

It is amazing how much you can progress week after week, month after month, year after year if you allow for gradual training increases.
— Bob Glover, *The Runner's Handbook*

⟨⧫⟩

If you under-train, you may not finish, but if you over-train, you may not start.
— Stan Jensen

When I was a customer service representative for a bank the year before the 1988 Olympics, I had to make time to run: before I went to work, on my lunch hour, and after work. It was no easy task, but the results were great.
—Florence Griffith Joyner

The more I train, the more I realize I have more speed in me.
—Leroy Burrell

I looked at Paavo Nurmi and the rest of the great Finnish runners before the war, and I realized that what set them up, apart from the others of the day, was that they did high mileage.
—Arthur Lydiard

Run like hell and get the agony over with.
—Clarence DeMar

When you first get a hill in sight, look at the top of it only once. Then imagine yourself at the bottom of the other side.
—Florence Griffith Joyner

Running was supposed to collapse my uterus.

    —Kathrine Switzer on an old wives' tales about why she shouldn't run

—◆—

Once upon a time, about twenty years ago to be precise, runners believed they didn't have to do anything but run.

    —Amby Burfoot, *The Principles of Running*

—◆—

What I was doing in the past was running my easy days too fast and not letting the body rest a bit, and then getting on the track and not putting in the times and the effort. And I was not fresh enough to enjoy what I was doing.

    —Priscilla Welch

—◆—

Fitness is like the blade of a knife; you want to sharpen it without ruining the blade.

    —Sally Jenkins, the *Washington Post*

—◆—

Coming from a farming background, I saw nothing out of the ordinary in running barefoot, although it seemed to startle the rest of the athletics world. I have always enjoyed going barefoot and when I was growing up I seldom wore shoes, even when I went into town.

    —Zola Budd

For me, a seven-minute-a-mile pace is fast enough, and I often run slower. I'll sometimes start a workout running an eight-minute or nine-minute pace. You can achieve a lot with slow workouts.

  —Doug Kurtis

———◆———

In running it is man against himself, the cruelest of opponents. The other runners are not the real enemies. His adversary lies within him, in his ability with brain and heart to master himself and his emotions.

  —Glenn Cunningham, American runner in the 1930s. He was
  severely burned in childhood and almost lost his legs.

———◆———

Racing teaches us to challenge ourselves. It teaches us to push beyond where we thought we could go. It helps us find out what we are made of.

  —Patti Sue Plumer, American Olympian in the 1992 Olympics

———◆———

We all have dreams. But in order to make dreams come into reality, it takes an awful lot of determination, dedication, self-discipline, and effort.

  —Jesse Owens

I have a resistance toward running.
    —Christy Turlington

If I can get better, why not?
    —Emil Zatopek

When you're young and training two or three times a day, you can beat every-body your age, but you'll only last a few years.
    —Arturo Barrios

[The athlete] must believe that through training his perfomance will improve and continue to improve indefinitely for as long as he continues to train to pro-gressively stiff standards.
    —Franz Stampfl

Mental toughness can take you to the top, and mental weakness straight to the bottom.
    —John Schiefer

Every so often, if you find your times slowing down, if you find your strength leaving you a little bit, don't try to push through it. Totally detrain.
—Priscilla Welch

——◆——

Leave your watch on the kitchen table and go—freely, like a child.
—Claire Kowalchik, *The Complete Book of Running for Women*

——◆——

You train best where you are the happiest.
—Frank Shorter

——◆——

I don't train. I just run my 3 to 15 miles a day.
—Jack Foster

——◆——

Races always evoke some dread about pain that will come. But we can't escape the fact that the more discomfort we accept in a race, the faster we will run. Successful racing means *courting the pain*.
—John Elliott

My basic philosophy can be summed up by an expression we use in Norwegian: hurry slowly. Get there, but be patient.
　　　　—Grete Waitz, *Run Your First Marathon*

Never really give in as long as you have an earthly chance.
　　　　—Alf Shrubb

If the ancient men ran, then so did ancient women. Atalanta was left to die in the forest by a cruel father who had wanted a son. The babe was suckled by a bear. A hunter saw her racing through the wilderness and was astonished by her beauty and speed.
　　　　—Benjamin Cheever, *Strides*

Many statistics say we only use a small percentage of our brains. I think the same can be said about the body.
　　　　—Peter Martins and New York City Ballet, *New York City Ballet Workout*

I learned, one, you shouldn't ever quit. And I learned, two, you'll never be able to explain it to anybody.
　　　　—Jim Ryun

Most people never run far enough on their first wind to find out they've got a second. Give your dreams all you've got and you'll be amazed at the energy that comes out of you.

—William James

When we run, we are already so exposed, often nearly naked in our shorts and T-shirts, huffing and puffing, purified by the effort. Briefly removed from the defenses and secrets we maintain in so much of our lives, we feel less need to hide our private thoughts, loves, fears, and stresses. We share.

—Amby Burfoot, *The Runner's Guide to the Meaning of Life*

Never attempt to pass a man on a bend, always improve your position on the straight.

—Harry Andrews

The man who can drive himself further once the effort gets painful is the man who will win.

—Roger Bannister

You need great humility to run a marathon!
—Grete Waitz and Gloria Averbuch, *Run Your First Marathon*

———◆———

Success is the result of the application of scientific methods of training to the development of natural talents or skill, which we all possess in some degree or another.
—Walter George

———◆———

I never had technique.
—Al Oerter

———◆———

Running on an artificial leg at full speed is like driving backward at 55 miles per hour, using only your rearview mirror to guide you.
—Thomas Bourgeois

———◆———

We train through the winter in deep snow and ice. Our slogan is "Pain is good, more pain is even better."
—Matt Carpenter, mountain runner

Pain, like time, is a backdrop to running.
　　　　—Sally Pont

Accept the ups and downs you will experience. You are going to have days you feel like you're flying and days you struggle. This is normal for all runners.
　　　　—Grete Waitz and Gloria Averbuch, *Run Your First Marathon*

I see elegance and beauty in every female athlete. I don't think being an athlete is unfeminine. I think of it as a kind of grace.
　　　　—Jackie Joyner-Kersee

Now, how would you define a track athlete who spends all of his or her time training and competing, is paid to appear in meets, paid bonuses for good performances, paid to wear certain shoes, paid to say good things about corporate sponsors? Unless you are totally naïve and incredibly ignorant, or unless you have reason to twist the truth, "professional" would have to be your answer.
　　　　—Carl Lewis

Set aside a time solely for running. Running is more fun if you don't have to rush though it.

    —Jim Fixx

<hr />

Track and field is not ice-skating. It is not necessary to smile and make a wonderful impression on the judges.

    —Emil Zatopek

<hr />

I have a good time. I let my mind go blank.

    —Jim Ryun

<hr />

I've learned that it's what you do with your miles, rather than how many you've run.

    —Rod DeHaven

CHAPTER FOUR

Our "Gigantic" running miscellany

Running with the Pack, Part I

Growing up as competitive athletes, we become inspired by great athletes who preceded us in the sport. The champion who inspired me most was one of the greatest, though his numerous world records long have been broken: Emil Zatopek of Czechoslovakia. Times aside, nobody has matched Zatopek's achievements, particularly at the 1952 Olympic Games when he won the 5,000 and 10,000 meters and the marathon.

As a middling runner at a small school in Minnesota (Carleton College), I read of the great Czech athlete's victories in *Track & Field News* and knew I never could attain the same level of glory.

Three years later, stationed with the U.S. Army in Germany, I attended a track meet in Furth featuring as its star performer Emil Zatopek, my hero. I was then not fast enough to receive an invitation to compete, so I hung on the fence surrounding the track to get as close as possible to the Czech as he effortlessly defeated a German opponent.

Each running step for the next year was run in pursuit of Emil Zatopek, not in expectation that I might beat him, but that I might narrow the time gap between us.

As chance would have it, the following summer I ran a 5,000 in Finland won by Zatopek the previous year. Much faster because of a year's hard training, I won though in inferior time. I had not defeated Emil Zatopek, but I was part of the chase pack.

Every one of the exceptional athletes quoted and mentioned in this chapter had a hero that propelled him or her in their training. We all run in the footsteps of those who were great before our time

An object at rest tends to stay at rest and an object in motion tends to stay in motion. . .
>   —Newton's first law of motion

Whatever the pace, run softly, run tall.
>   —Joe Henderson, *Running 101*

I was not very talented. My basic speed was low. Only with willpower was I able to reach this world-best standard in long-distance running.
>   —Emil Zatopek

Whatever moves the other runners made, I knew I could respond.
>   —Grete Waitz

You're only a hamstring injury away from oblivion.
>   —Steve Jones

When I was growing up I wasn't inspired to be a marathoner. It wasn't even in a little girl's vocabulary.

  —Lorraine Moller

I was now running for the tape, the mental agony of knowing I had hit my limit, of not knowing what was happening behind me. I was not to know they were fading, too.

  —Sebastian Coe

My goal was to figure out how I could win the Olympics. I had a plan and I trained with that goal in mind.

  —Lorraine Moller

This is what really matters: running. This is where I know where I am.

  —Steve Jones

When I am training and competing, I really concentrate, but during the rest of the day, I don't want to think about running.

  —Ingrid Kristiansen

Without some company in the difficult miles, the body's mission becomes lonely and dark.

  —Frank Shorter

I noted in my diary four or five things I did wrong in preparation for the race: like needing more 25-30 mile training runs, doing more speedwork, and drinking more fluids during a race. Unfortunately, I forgot all that at the Olympics.

  —Bill Rodgers on the 1976 Montreal Olympics

The marathon is my only girlfriend. I give her everything I have.

  —Toshihiko Seko

The only secret is that it is consistent, often monotonous, boring, hard work. And it's tiring.

  —Robert de Castella

It changed my life enormously. I had my head so firmly planted in the sand. Now I see how flimsy life is.

  —Priscilla Welch on her cancer diagnosis

Intercollegiate track meets were not very important. . . . He used them as speed work. . . . He used them as stepping stones to the marathon.
  —Bill Rodgers on Amby Burfoot

⊰•⊱

I keep on running figuratively and literally, despite a limp that gets more noticeable with each passing season, because for me there has always been a place to go and a terrible urgency to get there.
  —Joan Benoit Samuelson

⊰•⊱

I do everything I can to win.
  —Said Aouita

⊰•⊱

People who make mistakes in the early miles by going out too hard or by not taking enough water are the ones who aren't going to win the race, or, perhaps, even finish it.
  —Bill Rodgers

⊰•⊱

[O]f all the challenges I have faced, the greatest one has been the quest for combining my family and career.
  —Joan Benoit Samuelson

He taught us that the essence of running was picking apples, jumping in water, and that kind of stuff.
　　—Amby Burfoot on John Kelley

You can't rationalize performance.
　　—Frank Shorter

Even though I may have been a bit of a layabout and smoked and drank or whatever, I always worked for my money.
　　—Steve Jones

He wasn't expected to do well, and always ran like he had something to prove.
　　—Clive Thomas on Steve Jones

I deliberately kept a low profile, because then I could quietly go about my business and do what I knew how to do best.
　　—Lorraine Moller

He didn't have the marathon bug. He didn't have the focus he developed later.
—Amby Burfoot on Bill Rodgers in college

———◆———

My career coincided with the evolution of women's distance running. I was able to get on at the beginning of it and ride it right through.
—Lorraine Moller on her early running career

———◆———

He was the first to transform the 5,000 and 10,000 into a protracted sprint. That is how he felt he was his best. Because before Lasse, nobody ever went that early.
—Frank Shorter on how Lasse Viren changed racing tactics

———◆———

I never walked anywhere, it seems. I had a genuine, instinctive love of running.
—Sebastian Coe

———◆———

An athlete to a great extent determines his own training by his response to the tasks you set for him and by his racing results. The coach must adjust to his athlete.
—Peter Coe on training his son, Sebastian Coe

Carlos was the best in the world, but he was not always at his best. He wasn't always consistent.

  —Steve Jones on Carlos Lopes

———◆———

When I was a little girl, my parents said studying was the most important thing. "You need your job in the future, not sport," they told me. They couldn't believe running would be such a big thing for me.

  —Uta Pippig

———◆———

When you feel like going, wait for a couple of miles. And when you want to go again, wait for another couple of miles. Then, when you're ready again, wait for a couple more minutes.

  —Charlie Spedding's running advice to Steve Jones

———◆———

I remember watching Frank Shorter in the [1972 Munich Olympic] marathon. But I wasn't thinking that I'd end up in the Olympics. It was so far away from that, and something I couldn't conceive of.

  —Bill Rodgers

Your body follows the directives of the mind. Racing is such a direct feedback system that whatever thoughts you are holding are immediately represented in your body.

  —Lorraine Moller

———◆———

Doing something for yourself like running, and using it to test yourself, will only make you feel better about your career or your family role.

  —Joan Benoit Samuelson

———◆———

He runs like a man who's just been stabbed in the heart.

  —A coach on Emil Zatopek

———◆———

He runs with the grace of a bag thrown off the back of a mail truck. Somehow he finds the will to win.

  —Hal Higdon on Alberto Salazar

———◆———

For me it's the same, altitude or not.

  —Said Aouita on training in Boulder, Colorado

Ahh, once I was entered, I tried to win. I came in second.
>   —Emil Zatopek on his first race, which he tried to get out of by
>   playing sick.

———>•<———

Mr. Rodgers, you have to decide which is more important, your vocation or your avocation.
>   —School principal to Bill Rodgers

———>•<———

I've been trying to push it too far, but when you get to be 47 you start to think that time's not all before you, that you're not getting any younger, and there's a last-minute panic trying to cram everything in before the Big Curtain comes down.
>   —Priscilla Welch

———>•<———

He let the pack take him to 19 miles at perfect pace and he then found himself in the right place at the right time to move into the history books with an eyeballs-out, lung-busting, gut-wrenching six-mile surge to the finish.
>   —Charlie Spedding on Steve Jones's world record at the 1984 Chicago
>   Marathon

They are the people I work with and get my hands dirty with. They could relate to me because I'm just Steve to them, not someone like Sebastian Coe or Steve Cram.

> —Steve Jones on his friends and colleagues

⇒◆⇐

The Boston Marathon was his solitary goal. He put everything he had into it.

> —Bill Rodgers on Amby Burfoot

⇒◆⇐

Numbers don't lie. You always seem to remember your workouts as being a little better than they were. It's good to go back and review what you do.

> —Frank Shorter

⇒◆⇐

I lost my anonymity forever.

> —Grete Waitz on the consequences of winning the 1978
> New York City marathon

⇒◆⇐

[Lorraine] runs like a race horse, and I mean that as a compliment. She has these loping strides.

> —Marty Cooksey on Lorraine Moller

[Y]ou never know what can happen during a jog around the block or a 5-mile run.
—Florence Griffith Joyner

�------⟶

It sort of forces you to do it, because you don't want to let the other person down.
—Gordon Bakoulis on running with a partner

⟨------⟩

My whole teaching in one sentence is: "Run slowly, run daily, drink moderately, and don't eat like a pig."
—Dr. Ernest van Aaken, German physician and running coach

⟨------⟩

The average American takes twenty years to get out of condition and he wants to get back in condition in twenty days—and you just can't do it.
—Dr. Ken Cooper

⟨------⟩

I get more gratification out of getting some obese person who had a heart attack running around and enjoying life within a year. I get more gratification from that than putting a person in the Olympic games.
—Arthur Lydiard

There is no doubt that "Sport for All" is a twentieth century movement of real significance. Other mass movements have oppressed where they intended to liberate. This movement liberates because it has an essentially individual basis. The choice of speed, route, distance, or company is entirely yours.
    —Roger Bannister

I was tired from training and leading such a busy life, tired of having to bear the pressure and come through for others.
    —Grete Waitz on her decision to reduce her running in 1976

You may run faster tomorrow, but you won't run any bloody harder!
    —Percy Cerutty

Fear is a great motivator.
    —John Treacy

They stand near the line and pee on themselves. We always keep a mop near the start.
    —Fred Thompson on the six-year-olds at their first competition at
    New York's Colgate Games

I better go home before he breaks the rest of my records.
　　—Gunder Hagg, in the United States, when he heard that Arne
　　Andersson had broken his 1500m record back in Sweden

———⊰◈⊱———

Charlie had foregone running for the money. I had won money, but it just happened. That's not what I went to Chicago for.
　　—Steve Jones on Charlie Spedding

———⊰◈⊱———

God! He's running backwards!
　　—Broadcaster who saw Jim Peters collapse at the Empire Games
　　Marathon in 1954

———⊰◈⊱———

Great people and great athletes realize early in their lives their destiny, and accept it.
　　—Percy Cerutty

———⊰◈⊱———

I ran to get a letter jacket, a girlfriend.
　　—Jim Ryun

My parents had a certain idea of what they wanted their little girl to be and it did not include a budding track star.

 —Grete Waitz

———◆———

When I was small I was very naughty and my father chased me with his belt to give me a thrashing. Maybe that was how I got accustomed to running.

 —Fermin Cacho

———◆———

By a process of elimination, I went out for cross country.

 —Clarence DeMar

———◆———

At my school, I was timekeeper. It was my responsibility to make sure the other students were on time. So it was important that I arrived always first.

 —Ibraham Hussein on running miles to school as a child in Kenya

———◆———

In those school races, I always ran my legs off. There were girls watching and I wanted to impress them.

 —Juha Vaatainen

I know my going into running with a vengeance was to have something clear, definable, and precise.
　　　—Kenny Moore

I am just an athlete who can get fit for the right race at the right time.
　　　—Steve Jones

When I was 14 or 15, my brother tried to encourage me by giving me a pair of running shoes. But I threw them away because I was so used to running with bare feet and they were too heavy.
　　　—Haile Gebrselassie

I lost my first race at school and I was so jealous when the winner received a puppet that I said to myself, "I will carry on until I win a puppet."
　　　—Svetlana Masterkova

I look up to the five-minute milers. Because they don't get any of the good things I get. They're out there running just as hard.
　　　—Mark Belger

It was hard to find a pool when I was modeling in New York, so I took up running.

— Kim Alexis, supermodel

Sometimes people will say to me, "Oprah's got it easy because she's got a personal trainer and a personal chef." But that's baloney. No one can run for you. She was on the track every morning.

— Bob Greene, Oprah Winfrey's personal trainer

Music is my life, but running allows me to appreciate the music of the outdoors.

— Gail Williams, hornplayer

In every little village in the world there are great potential champions who only need motivation, development, and good exercise evaluation.

— Arthur Lydiard

I remember looking out the window and wondering what was out there and, now and then, I'd see a runner go by.

— Lorraine Moller on her hospitalization as a child

All I want to do is drink beer and train like an animal.
        —Rod Dixon

———◆———

I don't drink. I don't kiss girls. These things do an athlete in.
        —Suleiman Nyambui

———◆———

I am firmly of the impression that the athlete who indulges in an occasional glass of [beer] will, other things being equal, derive greater benefits thereby than the man who preserves and adheres to a rigid teetotalism.
        —Alf Shrubb

———◆———

My strength comes from my coach. Just as Alberto Salazar runs with God, I run with Coach Nakamura.
        —Toshihiko Seko

———◆———

Listen to your body. Do not be a blind and deaf tenant.
        —Dr. George Sheehan

Live like a clock.
  —Jumbo Elliott on how runners should arrange their days

———◆———

In my high school days, I found I couldn't defeat the other runners with speed, but I could on the distance side.
  —Bill Rodgers

———◆———

There is nothing more monotonous and sickening than running around a track.
  —Arthur Lydiard

———◆———

All top international athletes wake up in the morning feeling tired and go to bed feeling very tired.
  —Brendan Foster

———◆———

There's a lot to be said for LSD—long, slow distance, in this case.
  —Joe Henderson

I just want to make sure it's living hell for anyone out there who's going to beat me.

—Ken Souza on why he trains so hard

When I was living on my father's farm I used to run over obstacles all the time, chasing the cows and sheep.

—Moses Kiptauni on his childhood in Kenya

[H]e may have been king of the roads, but he was not regal, not chilly.

—Amby Burfoot on Bill Rodgers

I don't want to plead that it's the life of a monk, but I can't think of a sport—with the possible exception of swimming—where people train as hard.

—Sebastian Coe

The long run is what puts the tiger in the cat.

—Bill Squires

I had no idea of speedwork, so it was no wonder I remained a slow trudger for so many years!
  —Paavo Nurmi

—◆—

I say I'm going to finish last. That takes the pressure off.
  —Dan Middleman

—◆—

I found that working out in the morning helped get me going for the rest of the day, and working out in the afternoons helped relax me from a long day at the office.
  —Florence Griffith Joyner

—◆—

If you want to win a race you have to go a little berserk.
  —Bill Rodgers

—◆—

Road racing is rock 'n roll; track is Carnegie Hall.
  —Marty Liquori

After 5 or 6 laps I have read everyone like a newspaper and I know who is able to do this or that.
    —Miruts Yifter

I'm not a machine that can be wound up every day.
    —Herb Elliott

I think the idea of a two-hour marathon is thoroughly ridiculous. Absolutely ridiculous.
    —Derek Clayton

[D]on't be in a hurry, and never let any of the other runners know you are in a hurry even if you are.
    —Colin Smith

The struggle itself toward the heights is enough to fill man's heart. One must imagine Sisyphus happy.
    —Albert Camus

It is suicidal for other runners to copy my hill sessions without adequate backup.
—Pekka Vasala

————◆————

The victory took the stamp of eccentricity off me. I was a real athlete. My running had been looked upon as a diversion before.
—Frank Shorter on his 1972 Olympic Marathon win

————◆————

They are beautiful because they run and they run because they are beautiful.
—Dr. Ernest van Aaken when asked why beautiful women run

————◆————

In a country where only men are encouraged, one must be one's own inspiration.
—Tegla Loroupe, Kenya

————◆————

If this race is for "men only," why doesn't it say "men only" on the entry blank?
—Nina Kuscsik in 1969

People used to think I was a freak. Now women of all shapes and sizes run all the time. And they're not just beautiful and slim and wearing pink gossamer tights. They jiggle along at 12-minute miles or spring along at 6:30s. . . . That's what I love.

　—Kathrine Switzer

New York is the one you have to win.

　—Rod Dixon

I never felt as bad as I did over those last two miles. It was like running with a hangover.

　—Geoff Smith on the 1983 New York Marathon

I'm from Oregon, I hate New York, every day except Marathon Sunday.

　—Kenny Moore

Mind is everything: muscle—pieces of rubber. All that I am, I am because of my mind.

　—Paavo Nurmi

If I ever did what he did, I'd be dead from sheer exhaustion.
>>—Charlie Rodgers on his brother Bill

I don't know about psychology; I'm a runner.
>>—Steve Jones

The great thing about athletics is that it's like poker sometimes: you know what's in your hand and it may be a load of rubbish, but you've got to keep up the front.
>>—Sebastian Coe

Running is in my blood—the adrenaline flows before the races, the love/hate of butterflies in your stomach.
>>—Marcus O'Sullivan

I don't run for other people; I don't run for my country. I'm not very nationalistic. Derek Clayton comes first in my book.
>>—Derek Clayton

You could never get to talk to Nurmi. You could talk to the president of Finland, but not to Nurmi. He was a god.
—Arthur Lydiard

At least in a race you have mile markers and know how long you have to go. Labor is like running as hard as you can without knowing where the finish line is.
—Lorraine Moller on childbirth

The most important thing in the Olympic Games is not to win but to take part, just as the most important thing in life is not the triumph but the struggle.
—Baron de Coubertin, founder of the modern Olympics

⟨より⟩

You know, fourth is the absolutely worst place to finish in the Olympics.
—Eamonn Coghlan

⟨より⟩

People claim that fourth is the worst place to finish in the Olympics or Olympic Trials. Maybe, but I finished fifth in one Olympic Trials, and I much rather would have finished fourth.
—Hal Higdon

The Games are littered with people who had one good day and were never heard of or seen again.
  —Sebastian Coe

Remember, to be second behind Herb Elliott is like being an Olympic Champion.
  —Michel Jazy

Athletes should have the same opportunities as other artists and performers do, to perfect themselves through scholarships and fellowships to become artists in their sports.
  —Mario Moniz Pereira, Carlos Lopes's coach

We used to run just for the honor, for the glory, just to show people we could do it. The people run now because of the money involved, because of the contracts, because of the sponsors, etc.
  —Gaston Roelants

Medals are nice, but they are only symbols.
  —Emil Zatopek

I would rather not race many times for just money; I would rather win little bits of metal at the end of a colored ribbon.
— Charles Spedding

———⋖•◆•⋗———

If I had to choose between a gold medal and a happy family life, I'd take the good family life every time.
— Ron Clarke

———⋖•◆•⋗———

There's a lot of pressure to keep my record sparkling—no silvers or bronzes.
— Michael Johnson

———⋖•◆•⋗———

The day I retire is the day they drop me into the fire or burn me.
— Ron Hill

———⋖•◆•⋗———

Florence Griffith Joyner's contributions to society will undoubtedly last forever. Rarely do individuals possess the kind of strength, stability, and substance that took her from the ghetto of south-central Los Angeles to the White House in Washington, D.C.
— Jackie Joyner-Kersee on Florence Griffith Joyner

Some people can't live without booze; it looks like I can't live without running.
—Lasse Viren

———◆———

The athlete is another painter, another composer, another poet where the famous paintings, the sublime music, or the verses are replaced by world records. Athletics and running become a part of the story and tradition of the whole country in the future.
—Gunder Hagg

———◆———

If I faltered, there would be no arms to hold me and the world would be a cold and forbidding place.
—Roger Bannister

———◆———

It has such an historical significance, and it's such a big event, that, really, to win an Olympic medal for me is moving up into a new league. I'm in an exclusive club, something I have aspired to since I was a teenager.
—Lorraine Moller

———◆———

We can sprint the turn on a spring breeze and feel the winter leave our feet!
—Quentin Cassidy in John L. Parker Jr.'s *Once a Runner*

If everybody could get in on [running] on a world scale, it would really be hard for people to go to war.
—Ron Daws

It's just personal satisfaction.
—Kenny Moore

What used to be just a simple break-neck run when I was a little girl turned into some pretty technical training that involved a great deal of mental effort.
—Florence Griffith Joyner

I have to give up so many things, make so many personal sacrifices, to perform at my level, that I cannot even contemplate losing.
—Sebastian Coe

In the moment of victory I did not realize that the inner force, which had been driving me to my ultimate goal, died when I became the world's fastest miler.
—Derek Ibbotson in 1957

He had enough sense to back off when he needed to, and also was able to take on a lot of work.
    —Charlie Rodgers on his brother Bill

⋙◆⋘

It is very disappointing to lose in the last stride by the length of your nose.
    —Yevgeny Arzhanov

⋙◆⋘

Sometimes the difference between a good and a great runner is only an inch, as measured by exercise scientists. A good runner lifts two inches off the ground with each stride. A great runner rises only one inch, thus conserves energy.
    —Hal Higdon

⋙◆⋘

When I started running and competing at the age of 7, I had the worst form of anyone else running, and my coaches told me that if I wanted to improve my times, I had to improve my running form.
    —Florence Griffith Joyner

Bill was able to run a lot of races at a high level. I can think of only three runners who were able to do that: Bill, Juma Ikangaa, and Doug Kurtis.
—Frank Shorter on Bill Rodgers

❧

We didn't learn about anaerobic thresholds—simply the joy of running.
—Amby Burfoot on John Kelley

❧

If track is serious about ridding the sport of illegal drugs, then a separate organization is needed, whose only duty is to catch cheaters, regardless of the potential media impact.
—Steve Holman

❧

Hitler was there every day, watching. He looked like Charlie Chaplin sitting up there, him and that fat guy, Goering.
—John A. Kelly, on the 1936 Berlin Olympics

❧

Thrust against pain, pain is the purifier.
—Percy Cerutty

When I am running, I feel everything is in sync. Even my mechanical leg becomes a part of me.

—Sarah Reinersten

———◆———

Concentration is why some athletes are better than others. You develop that concentration in training. You can't be lackadaisical in training and concentrate in a meet.

—Edwin Moses

———◆———

I love buying running shoes. I don't mean that I just enjoy the process of trying on new shoes. I mean I love buying running shoes.

—John Bingham

CHAPTER FIVE

Triumph and tragedy

Running Races

All my marathon training programs peak at 20 miles. And among the most frequently asked questions asked me at lectures or posted to the bulletin boards I manage online is: "How can I expect to run 26 miles 385 yards when the furthest you let me run in practice is 20 miles?"

My glib answer is to suggest that a million-plus runners using my programs have taken that approach. "Have faith," I say.

But the truth is that before a marathon, or any other important race, runners will have rested. For a marathon, they taper three weeks. Even an important 5-K requires a cutback in training for three or four days if you expect to do your best. In contrast, that 20-mile run is completed after a hard week of work.

Before a race, runners eat right. They skip that extra beer or glass of wine the night before. They don't stay out late. They get to sleep early. When they step to the starting line the next morning, it is with a purpose, more than for just another day in practice. Once moving, the sounds of the crowd and the footsteps of their fellow competitors carry them along. Several top athletes quoted in this chapter talk about the "fear" of failure. I have never been able to run as fast in practice as I have in either a track meet or road race.

As for the marathon and why I recommend a longest run of only 20 miles, I consider the last 6 miles 385 yards to be sacred ground. You only dare enter with a number pinned to your chest.

Do otherwise, and the gods will be angry.

No matter how old I get, the race remains one of life's most rewarding experiences.
—George Sheehan

My thoughts before a big race are usually pretty simple. I tell myself: "Get out of the blocks, run your race, stay relaxed. If you run your race, you'll win. . . . Channel your energy. Focus."
—Carl Lewis

You hear it over and over again—a television announcer saying, "Watch that guy, he looks so relaxed." It's a rare athlete who wins who doesn't look relaxed.
—Mark Allen

When you put yourself on the line in a race and expose yourself to the unknown, you learn things about yourself that are very exciting.
—Doris Brown Heritage

A road race is the closest thing to a party I can think of.
—Bill Rodgers, *Bill Rodgers' Lifetime Running Plan*

There will come a point in the race, when you alone will need to decide. You will need to make a choice. Do you really want it? You will need to decide.
    —Rolf Arands

———✦———

Good health, peace of mind, being outdoors, camaraderie—those are all wonderful things that come to you when running. But for me, the real pull of running—the proverbial icing on the cake—has always been racing.
    —Bill Rodgers, *Bill Rodgers' Lifetime Running Plan*

———✦———

There is a world of difference between racing for time and racing to win. The white line and clear course are needed for one; generalship, ability to change pace, and track tactics for the other.
    —The *Daily Mirror*, June 4, 1954

———✦———

Some runners judge performance by whether they won or lost. Others define success or failure by how fast they ran. Only you can judge your performance. Avoid letting others sit in judgment of you.
    —Hal Higdon

Sex doesn't always determine who will be the fastest. . . . Look at any race and you'll see that the best women beat most of the men.
—Claire Kowalchik, *The Complete Book of Running for Women*

To make your life a work of art, you must have the material to work with. The race, any race, is just such an experience.
—George Sheehan

No one competes with the reckless abandon they should. . . . I'd personally rather watch someone who runs his guts out, throws his breakfast up and passes out at the end of the race.
—John Schiefer

Most mistakes in a race are made in the first two minutes, perhaps in the very first minute.
—Jack Daniels, Exercise Physiologist and Coach

Average runners often use racing as one of the goals in their training. Maybe it is to help them continue through their training, maybe it motivates them to get out there on a consistent basis.

—Frank Shorter

—❖—

You should not do more than two races a month if you want those races to be key, maximum efforts. . . . Otherwise, staleness and breakdown may occur.

—Cliff Held

—❖—

If I do well in a race I'm to the moon. If I do exceptionally well, I've jumped over that moon.

—Priscilla Welch

—❖—

To avoid starting out too fast, you have to "have eyes in your stomach," as we say in Norwegian: a good gut instinct of control.

—Grete Waitz

Inevitably, there's some official bellowing: "Come on! Run through the chute! Keep it movin'!" But you're bent over, gasping, admiring with salt-stung eyes the good, honest mud of battle . . . splattered on your still-quivering legs and too-old (but still lucky) racing shoes. What could be more beautiful?
—Mark Will-Weber

My whole feeling in terms of racing is that you have to be very bold. You sometimes have to be aggressive and gamble.
—Bill Rodgers

The agony of the runners was a visible, tangible thing. It was only courage and the deepest reserves of stamina that were driving them round the track, still competing, still fighting it out.
—William R. Loader, "Staying the Distance"

There is something about the ritual of the race—putting on the number, lining up, being timed—that brings out the best in us.
—Grete Waitz

Fear is probably the thing that limits performance more than anything—the fear of not doing well, of what people will say. You've got to acknowledge those fears, then release them.

 —Mark Allen

———

Foley knew the dread of the slow minutes before a race begins—the draw for the positions, the bumbling instructions from judge and starter, the final hush when the starter's commands begin: "On your marks!"

 —Eddy Orcutt, "Wheelbarrow"

———

[I]n athletics, the main essence is races, races against opponents, more than against the clock. . . . And those will be what I shall set my main sights on.

 —Roger Bannister

———

I'm going to go and leave my blood all over the track.

 —Nick Rogers, Olympian

I made the school team, and when I won in a match against another school it was the greatest moment of my life—even greater than the European titles. In those school races, I always ran my legs off. There were girls watching and I wanted to impress them. I was foaming and vomiting, but I won.
　　　　—Juha Väätäinen

It wasn't enough for me to win the race. I wanted to bury the other guys.
　　　　—Alberto Salazar

In the field of sports, you are more or less accepted for what you do rather than what you are.
　　　　—Althea Gibson

Strategy-wise, go with your strengths. If you don't have a great finish, you must get away to win.
　　　　—John Treacy

In any race there are the moments you feel great, and the moments you feel you're not going to make it.
　　　　—Mark Allen

You have your own strategy and what you do is go out and use it, and structure the situation so everyone else is forced to use your strategy . . . it really is a control issue.
—Frank Shorter

———⟫◆⟪———

I felt my throat start to close up, and I didn't think I was getting enough oxygen. I was scared, and I thought about quitting. But you don't want to quit when you've trained so hard and long for one race.
> —Deena Drossin describing the effects of being stung by a bee in the back of the throat 100 meters after the start of the World Cross-Country Championships in Portugal. Despite blacking out and falling during the 8k race, she finished in twelfth place.

———⟫◆⟪———

The most challenging aspect of the decathlon is not the events themselves, but how you train to become the best 100-meter runner you are on the same day that you're the best 1,500-meter runner.
—Bruce Jenner

———⟫◆⟪———

Blink and you miss a sprint. The 10,000 meters is lap after lap of waiting. Theatrically, the mile is just the right length—beginning, middle, end: a story unfolding.
—Sebastian Coe

Some of the world's greatest feats were accomplished by people not smart enough to know they were impossible.
　　　—Doug Larson

If you want to race and get the best possible results, choose races carefully and focus on them.
　　　—Francie Larrieu Smith

I don't want to lose to no one.
　　　—Gabe Jennings

I ran my first sub-4-minute mile in 1977 and since then have run 136 more. Nobody has run as many sub-4s as I have, and I intend to run at least one more.
　　　—Steve Scott, after cancer surgery

The 800-meter record, the records in the 1000, the 1500, the 5000, the relays: no one remembers them. The mile, they remember. Only the mile.
　　　—John Walker

The mile has all the elements of drama.
  —Roger Bannister

———◆———

Almost every part of the mile is tactically important: you can never let down, never stop thinking, and you can be beaten at almost any point. I suppose you could say it is like life.
  —John Landy

———◆———

I've always found it effective to make a move just before the crest of a hill. You get away just a little and you're gone before your opponent gets over the top.
  —John Treacy

———◆———

Jogging through the forest is pleasant, as is relaxing by the fire with a glass of gentle Bordeaux and discussing one's travels. Racing is another matter. The frontrunner's mind is filled with an anguished fearfulness, a panic, which drives into pain.
  —Kenny Moore

No one knows the fear in a frontrunner's mind more than me. When you set off at a cracking pace for four or five laps and find that your main rivals are still breathing down your neck, that's when you start to panic.
—Ron Clarke

—◆—

He cleared the hurdles like he feared they had spikes imbedded on the top, and leaped the water hazard as if he thought crocodiles were swimming in it.
—Description of Kenya's Amos Biwotts

—◆—

I eat whatever the guy who beat me in the last race ate.
—Alex Ratelle

—◆—

Whether we athletes liked it or not, the 4-minute mile had become rather like an Everest: a challenge to the human spirit, it was a barrier that seemed to defy all attempts to break it, an irksome reminder that men's striving might be in vain.
—Roger Bannister

—◆—

The athlete knows he controls what happens to him. He blames no one but himself when things go wrong.
—George Sheehan

I haven't run as fast as I can, I haven't spoken as well as I can, and I haven't written as well as I can. If you take any less than that view, you're finished.

    —George Sheehan

———◆———

These high, wild hills and rough, uneven ways draw out our miles and make them wearisome.

    —Shakespeare, *Richard II*

———◆———

I'd rather run a gutsy race, pushing all the way and lose, than run a conservative race only for a win.

    —Alberto Salazar

———◆———

You have to forget your last marathon before you try another. Your mind can't know what's coming.

    —Frank Shorter

———◆———

Everyone stumbles at one time or another. It's the human condition.

    —Amby Burfoot, *The Runner's Guide to the Meaning of Life*

Several times I have been threatened with overthrow by phenomenals. On one or two occasions it has been whispered around in such a way as to reach my ears, that importations have been made and it was goodbye to Shrubb. These importations have once or twice materialized. Like deer they would run for a distance and keep me guessing. All of a sudden they would disappear and I, smilingly relieved, would trudge on alone.

—Alf Shrubb

CHAPTER SIX

Keeping pace with the "elites"

Front Runners

The day before the Boston Marathon one year, I went for a short run on the banks of the Charles River, across the expressway, not far from the hotels where most runners stay. I was in Boston as a reporter, not as a runner, but I wanted to identify with those who would toe the starting line in Hopkinton the next day. So I ran from my hotel to the river, a distance of about a mile. I stopped. I stretched, lying down on the grass on a warm day to do so. Then I jogged back toward my hotel at a very slow pace befitting someone whose best competitive days were well behind him.

Ahead, I spied three Kenyan runners returning to their hotel from a different direction. Using a pedestrian walkway, they crossed the expressway before I reached it. Then as we continued up a slight incline toward Boylston Street, I found that I was catching them! I could not pass. That would be an assault on reality, so I slowed and allowed the talented trio to reach the hotel before me.

Some people think that Kenyans always run fast, that every stride is at a pace near 90 percent of maximum. Not true. Like most successful elite runners, they know when to push, and they know when to rest.

The next time I saw the three Kenyans was from the press truck during the Boston Marathon. They were leading the race.

ROGER BANNISTER

I was startled and frightened. I glanced round uneasily to see if anyone was watching. A few more steps—self-consciously . . . the earth seemed almost to move with me. I was running now, and a fresh rhythm entered my body.
>—Roger Bannister on first running when he was a child

If there was a moment when things began, that was it for me.
>—Roger Bannister on watching Arne Andersson beat Sydney
>Wooderson at a track meet in 1945

I'm afraid that you'll never be any good. You just haven't got the strength or build for it.
>—Oxford groundskeeper to Roger Bannister on running

A hard-working medical student who between writing theses and delivering babies, turns his brain to the technique and theory of running.
>—The *Daily Telegraph*

We heard wonderful stories in Helsinki that Bannister would win because he had done a world-shattering time in a secret trial before leaving. MAYBE HE DID. ANYONE CAN RUN QUICKLY PAST TREES!

  —The *Daily Mirror* on Bannister's failure at the Helsinki Olympics

A disaster is something which is shared between you and the public which expects something of you and which you cannot or have not fulfilled.

  —Roger Bannister on the 1952 Helsinki Olympics, where he did not
  run well

Bannister had terrific grace, a terrific long stride, he seemed to ooze power. It was as if the Greeks had come back and brought to show you what the true Olympic runner was like.

  —*Daily Mail* journalist Terry O'Connor

Anyone who beats him in the Olympics at Helsinki will have to fly.

  —British official

Bannister has a fine, though by no means an inordinately strong physique. Many others have been as richly blessed as he. His running is a triumph of technique . . . and his success is the result of applying his intellect to the job.

—The *Daily Telegraph*

To say . . . "Four minutes is only a time" was presumptuous, unless I had an answer for the inevitable follow-up question—"Well, if it's possible, why don't you do it?"

—Roger Bannister on questions from the press

Roger, you only become really friendly with your opponents after you've beaten them!

—Don Macmillan to Roger Bannister

There are times the night before a race when he actually makes involuntary sounds, like a man being tortured. Roger is a hard man to comfort—if you try, he'll give you a look that goes right through you.

—Chris Chataway

Sport is about not being wrapped up in cotton wool.
 —Roger Bannister

⟞◆⟝

Sport is about adapting to the unexpected and being able to modify plans at the last minute.
 —Roger Bannister

⟞◆⟝

I knew you would do it one day, Roger.
 —Roger Bannister's mother after he broke the four-minute mile in 3:59.4 on May 6, 1954

⟞◆⟝

It is in fact only a time.
 —Roger Bannister

⟞◆⟝

No words could be invented for such supreme happiness.
 —Roger Bannister on breaking the four-minute mile

ARTURO BARRIOS

Go knock on Arturo Barrios's door. If I was a young runner today, I'd go and hang around with the top guys like Arturo, and see what he is doing.
> —Frank Shorter's advice to young runners

JOSEY BARTHEL

He had had no trainer and no compatriot with him when he came into the stadium, and he was still alone. It must have been a great solace to him on the night before the race, knowing he had nobody to disappoint.
> —A. J. Liebling on Josey Barthel at the 1952 Helsinki Olympics.
> Barthel won the 1,500-meter event.

DICK BEARDSLEY

It's not really bragging if you back it up.
> —Dick Beardsley

———✦———

Holy shit, Dickie! You're leading the New York City Marathon!
> —Bill Squires

———✦———

Dick was our sport's best-known "good guy." Everyone in the running community liked Dick.
> —Bill Rodgers

Some of those kids come to you, they look like guppies. You wanna say, "Come on, kid, go buy some roller skates, get lost." But Dickie wasn't like that. You could tell that underneath all that aw-shucks crap he was tough as nails.
—Bill Squires

———

When I see a videotape of the race, I think of how much fun it would have been to attend as a spectator . . . just to watch. Let alone be in it. Even watching a tape today, it makes the hair on the back of my neck stand up.
—Dick Beardsley on his famous race against Alberto Salazar

———

Every marathon I ran, I knew I had a faster one in me.
—Dick Beardsley

———

He might as well have told me I was pregnant, that's how much trouble I had believing this was happening.
—Dick Beardsley on when Bill Squires agreed to coach him

We start talking workouts, and he wants to show me his training log. I said, "Jesus Christ, I don't wanna read that thing. The only thing I read is the obituaries in the morning paper to see if I'm still alive."

—Bill Squires on coaching Beardsley

———⟫◆⟪———

It was so thick with spectators you couldn't even see how the hills went up. It was just this mass of humanity, people hanging out of trees or whatever.

—Dick Beardsley on the Boston Marathon crowds

———⟫◆⟪———

Dickie had the most beautiful, efficient style I ever saw. When you watched Dickie run, violins played and little birdies flew around.

—Bill Squires

———⟫◆⟪———

Neither of us ran this well again. We didn't give an inch, and about killed each other in the process. Seriously. I was never the same again, running, mentally or physically.

—Dick Beardsley on his famous race against Alberto Salazar

———⟫◆⟪———

I've never been the slightest bit bored with running.

—Dick Beardsley

You better be careful, Dick. You're playing with fire by running so many fast marathons. The body's not designed for that kind of stress. Sooner or later you're going to have to pay a price.

—Garry Bjorklund

———✦———

Sooner or later, someone always asks about the '82 Boston. I don't mind—I like talking about it, and so does Dick. That's because we never discuss the race in terms of running a 2:08 or beating the other guy. It took us both a long, long time, but we finally realized that that's not what the marathon is really about.

—Alberto Salazar

———✦———

I ran the race of my life, 2:08:53. Alberto happened to run two seconds faster. All I know for certain is that I left everything I had out on that course. I didn't give an inch. Neither did Alberto. The way I look at it, there were two winners that day.

—Dick Beardsley

ABEBE BIKILA

Abebe planted the idea that the marathon could be raced in a different way. Up until then, people would save themselves, waiting to see who would drop. He helped change the tactics.

—Frank Shorter

GARRY BJORKLUND

It's not uncommon to come across a cross-country runner; it's not uncommon to come across a track runner; and it's not uncommon to come across a road runner. But to find that mix of all three is special.

—Garry Bjorklund

❦

As they prepare you to go out onto the track, you walk through a labyrinth of tunnels. You don't actually see the track until they lead you out. We sat in a room beneath the stadium, where they checked our spikes and numbers, and we could hear the pulsing of the crowds outside, reverberating. We could feel the Olympics, but not see them.

—Garry Bjorklund on the Olympics

BILL BOWERMAN

He tailored our training to the peculiarities of our talents. When he made me take extra days of rest between workouts, I improved so much it was an epiphany.

—Kenny Moore

❦

Bowerman was the guide or teacher who appears in every mythic narrative at Oregon about coming of age. His main lesson was, in the words of the oracle, "Know thyself."

—Kenny Moore

CHRIS BRASHER

You had the feeling that he wanted to master what he was doing and literally forced himself to do it.

> —A friend

CHRIS CHATAWAY

Both were as fresh as paint at the finish.

> —AAA National Coach Geoffrey Dyson after watching Bannister
> and Chataway race

———◆———

He's the one who makes me work—and keeps me amused. He will soon run a four-minute mile himself.

> —Roger Bannister

EAMONN COGHLAN

I do love to run indoors. I love the tightness of the track. . . . The crowd is right on top of you.

> —Eamonn Coghlan

That magical four-minute mile barrier has set a universal standard. To run under that time is a phenomenal achievement. For the average runner, to see how close that person can come to the "almighty" gives them an indication of where they really stand.
—Eamonn Coghlan

In certain ways, the feeling of running a mile in 3:49 is exactly the same as when I ran my first marathon in 2:25 in New York in 1991. And that sheer exhilaration that you experience is the same for a world-class runner as it is for a jogger.
—Eamonn Coghlan

Running a fast mile feels almost like you're flying like a bird, in complete control of everything that's going on, physically and mentally. You feel absolutely fantastic, like a runaway express train that could effortlessly go on and on forever.
—Eamonn Coghlan

I think everyone should try running a mile. People can relate to the mile.
—Eamonn Coghlan

BILL EASTON

We never run a race we don't figure we can win. If you don't feel that way, why run?
>   —Bill Easton on his team

⬥

"Merry Christmas! . . . Be ready for hard workouts upon your return to the campus."
>   —Bill Easton's 1953 Christmas card to his team at the University of
>   Kansas

HERB ELLIOTT

It was just another time, another progression.
>   —Herb Elliott after running a 3:54.5 mile in 1958

HAILE GEBRSELASSIE

Haile Gebrselassie is the best distance runner I have seen in the last quarter century, the most electrifying personality, and somewhat of an enigma, given his Ethiopian roots.
>   —Amby Burfoot

⬥

Be in no doubt Haile is the greatest distance runner the world has ever seen.
>   —Dave Bedford

Haile is an elegant champion and a fine example of sportsmanship.
　　—Lasse Viren

It makes you want to quit.
　　—Mark Plaatjes on Haile Gebrselassie's record times

One gold medal in a championship is ordinary. I wanted to get two golds and be a little different.
　　—Haile Gebreselassie

FLORENCE GRIFFITH JOYNER

We entered a new era with Flo-Jo on the scene, particularly for women. She was dynamic out there, very sophisticated. She put a new twist on women's competitive sports.
　　—USA Track and Field President Patricia Rico

There's a very short list of instantly recognizable female athletes. Flo-Jo is one of those athletes.
　　—Bob Williams

She's been an inspiration for a lot of young women and men also. She has tried to give back to inner-city kids.

> —400-meter hurdler Sandra Farmer Patrick

—◈—

Sadly, her life has passed as rapidly as her races.

> —Primo Nebiolo, head of track and field's world governing body
>   IAAF

—◈—

Florence Griffith Joyner was one of a kind. She did many different things with style and grace.

> —Bert Rosenthal

—◈—

She just had so much style and grace and inward and outward beauty.

> —Sandra Farmer Patrick

—◈—

Florence brought a certain style to the track, something so different, with her fashionable appearance and her stunning speed.

> —Patricia Rico

Her legacy will be one that includes kindness and interest in children and their dreams.
　　—Bill Hybl

It takes practice and perseverance, but as long as I hold on to my dreams, I know they'll become a reality.
　　—Florence Griffith Joyner

KIP KEINO

When Henry Rono was a young boy, Kipchoge Keino gave a talk in a stadium near Eldoret, Kenya. Rono did not go in. Instead he climbed a tree and watched the Olympian Keino talk to the crowd. Up in the tree Rono vowed he would one day be as great a runner as Keino.
　　—Michael Sandrock

He was a mystery. There was an aura of invincibility about him.
　　—Frank Shorter

He was a competitor in his whole lifestyle.
　　—Mal Whitfield

Sometimes I win and sometimes I don't. The cap has nothing to do with it. The race is in God's hands.

  —Kip Keino, answering reporters' questions on whether his orange
   hat had any sort of significance

———⊷◆⊶———

Kipchoge was a natural. He did what he was born to do. He grew up in a good traditional society, with natural living. He didn't dissipate his energy, but stayed focused on who and what he wanted to become.

  —Mal Whitfield

———⊷◆⊶———

People really feared him when he was running.

  —Frank Shorter

———⊷◆⊶———

I think a big enemy for world-ranking African athletes like Keino is their generous nature and the readiness to run anywhere any time.

  —Peter Snell

One of the athletes I admired most was Kip Keino, who was a real gentleman, highly intelligent, and a brilliant runner, so versatile. He was one of the founders of the great Kenyan distance-running history.
—Arthur Lydiard

When my father started out, he wasn't so good. He realized he could be good after he got some international exposure and was fifth in the [1964] Olympics. That's when he increased his training and that's when he got good.
—Martin Keino

He wasn't cocky after he won; he was just a natural, and he was always humble.
—Mal Whitfield

JOHNNY KELLEY

I think the job toughened me up, climbing and walking and stooping all day. When I began my run at night, I was tired; but after a mile or so, the tiredness went away.
—Three-time Boston Marathon winner Johnny Kelley on his job at Boston Edison Electric Company

JOHN LANDY

While you were at the pictures, or square dancing, last Saturday night, John Landy was doing a 10-mile training run.

—Harry Hopman in the *Melbourne Herald*

———◆———

I just go out there and work. I've got to punish myself to get anywhere.

—John Landy to the *Sydney Morning Herald*

———◆———

A certain amount of nervous energy to be released. . . . A level track with "life" in it.

—Frank Tierney in the *Sydney Morning Herald* on two of the
conditions John Landy would need in order to break the four-
minute mile

———◆———

There is no gray—just black and white. . . . If you're hurt enough to limp, you can't run at all. If you aren't, it makes no difference.

—John Landy to *Sports Illustrated*

[Running] teaches you the ability to present under pressure.
  —John Landy

***

[Running] teaches you the importance of being enthusiastic, dedicated, focused.
  —John Landy

***

Landy had tried so hard, and I am very glad that he has now succeeded. It shows that times can always be broken.
  —Roger Bannister after Landy beat his mile record, running a 3:58
   time

***

It was done. Finished. Next thing.
  —John Landy on his attitude after running a 3:58 mile

***

I can do even better.
  —John Landy

CARL LEWIS

After I left the podium in Atlanta, I felt so fulfilled in my career that I lost my desire to compete at that level again.

—Carl Lewis, after the Atlanta Olympics

———⟶◆⟵———

Trust funds are not necessary anymore. They give the public a false impression that the athletes somehow are still amateur.

—Carl Lewis

JOHN LODWICK

It was a tremendous amount of work and a tremendous amount of fun.

—John Lodwick on his years as a professional runner for Nike's Athletics West team

———⟶◆⟵———

I was extremely serious about running, obviously, but I primarily thought of it as a way to know and serve God. For me, running was a way to witness.

—John Lodwick

We were young and single and caught up in something important—something that was much more than a sport.

> —John Lodwick on his years as a professional runner for Nike's Athletics West team

———

At times, at its best, running could even be a form of prayer.

> —John Lodwick

JACK LOVELOCK

It was all so easily accomplished, with so little outward evidence of stress and strain, as to make a four-minute mile seem just around the corner.

> —*The New York Herald Tribune* on Lovelock's 4:07.6 race on July 15, 1933

———

I have now learned better than to have my races dictated by the public and the press, so I did not throw away a certain championship merely to amuse the crowd and be spectacular.

> —Jack Lovelock, 1936 Olympic Gold Medalist

———

You mean *the* Jack Lovelock.

> —Roger Bannister when he met Lovelock in 1947

BILLY MILLS

Worry about him? I never even heard of him.

> —Ron Clarke, Australian distance runner, on Billy Mills's 10,000 victory in the Tokyo Olympics, 1964

———◆———

Coming off the last turn, my thoughts changed from 'One more try, one more try, one more try. . .' to 'I can win! I can win! I can win!'

> —Billy Mills

PAAVO NURMI

The Olympic Torch is being brought into the stadium by . . . P-A-A-V-O N-U-R-M-I.

> —Announcement at the 1952 Helsinki Olympics

———◆———

Once, it is said, he ran 40 miles from a small town to his home in Turku on the northwest coast of Finland. His wife heard a faint scratching on their back door. Thinking it was a neighborhood dog, she opened the door. There was Paavo, slumped in a heap on the doorstep, so exhausted from his run that he could not open the door.

> —Michael Sandrock

GORDON PIRIE

Pirie is the most extraordinary runner the world has known, bearing in mind his amazing type of training and the distances over which he seems to be able to beat records.

　　　—Joseph Binks

STEVE PREFONTAINE

At a very young age, he was competitive against the best in the world. He certainly wasn't scared of running against whomever.

　　　—Alberto Salazar on Steve Prefontaine

———◆———

To give anything less than your best is to sacrifice the gift.

　　　—Steve Prefontaine

———◆———

His talent was not that he had great style. He didn't. It got better, I think. We worked probably harder on that than we did on anything.

　　　—Walt McClure

———◆———

Pre inspired a whole generation of American distance runners to excel. He made running cool.

　　　—Alberto Salazar

I haven't seen too many American distance men on the international scene willing to take risks. I saw some U.S. women in Barcelona willing to risk, more than men. The Kenyans risk. Steve Prefontaine risked. I risked—I went through the first half of the Tokyo race just a second off my best 5000 time.

   —Billy Mills, gold medal winner of the 10,000 at the 1964 Tokyo
      Olympics with a 46-second PR.

<hr/>

The minute Pre hit the field for his jog, there was an undercurrent of enthusiasm in the crowd. It surfaced in slight cheers as he raced down the stretch. You could feel the electricity.

   —Geoff Hollister

<hr/>

I was really gung-ho the whole next year, 1972, trying to get into good enough shape to say, "I'm going to stick with the guy and possibly beat him in the end."

   —Greg Fredericks

<hr/>

He was self-confident, yes, sir. He wasn't cocky, as a lot of people accused him of later. He had a lot of pride, but it was constructive.

   —Walt McClure

To understand Steve Prefontaine, it is necessary to know something about Coos Bay, Oregon. The town and the man find themselves similarly described: blunt, energetic, tough, aggressive.
　　—Kenny Moore

<hr>

What I want is to be number one.
　　—Steve Prefontaine

<hr>

He wouldn't take second effort—it wasn't acceptable. It was all out. When you're like that, when you start doing that, you become a lot more consistent.
　　—Alberto Salazar

<hr>

He was always running up and down, shouting encouragement and advice. We finally had to tell him, "Look, we'll do the coaching, you do the running."
　　—Walt McClure

<hr>

A lady came into the store where I worked, and said, "Mrs. Prefontaine, you should go to the meets. Your son is Olympic stuff." I still remember the words.
　　—Steve Prefontaine's mother

I was standing on a hill. I had my binoculars, and I was probably a good half-mile or 700 yards away from the start. And I saw this guy that had the start position, but it was the look in his eyes from a half-mile distance, the intensity in his face as the gun went off. I thought, "That's got to be Pre."

  —Bill Dellinger on first seeing Steve Prefontaine

———◆———

What I like most about track is the feeling I get inside after a good run.

  —Steve Prefontaine

BILL RODGERS

The gun goes off and the next thing I know, we pass 10 miles in 50 minutes, and there's a runner next to me—it's Bill Rodgers. It was his first race in God knows how long, and he ran 1:47 something for 20 miles. I was surprised as could be.

  —Amby Burfoot on a 1973 race

———◆———

We were always moving. We'd go out and play in the woods, and I always had a lot of energy.

  —Bill Rodgers on his childhood

The coach would send us off on a long run—which then might be three miles—and Bill would be far more into it than me or the other guys. I'd take off and go to my girlfriend's house, but Bill would go run for an hour.
    —Charlie Rodgers, Bill's brother, on high school cross country days

---

[Running] was the only area of my life where I was successful.
    —Bill Rodgers

Billy was the man, and I was one of the guys who wanted to dethrone the king. It's to his credit that I had so many opportunities to try, and never did.
    —Garry Bjorklund

When I was fired, I had time on my hands. And it was gnawing at me psychologically to do something positive with my life.
    —Bill Rodgers

One of Bill's brilliant, brilliant things was that he returned every phone call from every journalist, meaning he was written up by every paper big and small.
    —Amby Burfoot

He just toys with fields. He plays with them. It's almost a joke.
—Tommy Leonard

———◆———

We'd go looking for butterflies, and sometimes it would get competitive, and I'd run and swoop them from under the noses of my friends.
—Bill Rodgers on his childhood

———◆———

I introduced my wife to Billy, and afterwards she just couldn't believe he was the king of the roads. She thought he was just a mild-mannered schoolteacher from suburban Boston. And he was—until he laced on his shoes.
—Garry Bjorklund

———◆———

Bill beat me like a drum. I never thought of it as personal rivalry but one from an athletic standpoint.
—Frank Shorter

———◆———

I'm just lucky in terms of the biomechanics. I've never had a broken bone or a sprained ankle.
—Bill Rodgers

He ran with a relaxed, flowing stride, and he seemed to have the ability to go out there and hammer people in the middle of the race and not leave it to the end.

  —Amby Burfoot

***

I don't feel quite so smooth when I'm running now, like I'm always running uphill or against a headwind. But I get inspired by progress, which is why I like running. You can always improve through your efforts.

  —Bill Rodgers in 1996

ALBERTO SALAZAR

If there are no injuries or unforeseen developments . . . well, the facts are plain; I'm the fastest man in the race.

  —Alberto Salazar before the 1982 Boston Marathon

***

I always claim that the marathon is just another race to me. But Billy [Bill Rodgers] insists that someday the marathon could humble you.

  —Alberto Salazar

I look at that marathon as the epitome of what running is all about.
　　—Alberto Salazar on the 1982 Boston Marathon

JOAN BENOIT SAMUELSON

All athletes who strive for excellence share the same story.
　　—Joan Benoit Samuelson

———◆———

I run. I am a runner. I am an athlete.
　　—Joan Benoit Samuelson

———◆———

In March, 1983, the Friday before the World Cross-Country Championships in Gateshead, England, Benoit took me on a 10-mile run. She picked it up until I was using everything I had to stay with her. Then, up a long English hill in the rain, she became the first woman ever to run away from me.
　　—Kenny Moore

———◆———

Women's running has come of age, thanks in great measure to the incomparable strides of Joan Samuelson.
　　—Kathrine Switzer

Joan is a world-class athlete in touch with the most important aspects of physical endurance and perseverance and of striving to realize a dream despite any obstacles.
—Gloria Averbuch

No athlete was ever tougher than Joan Benoit, and no one more defining in her cycle of injury, recovery, victory, and injury—of love and loving too much.
—Kenny Moore on Joan Benoit Samuelson

Even as Benoit won the first women's Olympic marathon in 1984, I knew she was a legend. . . . I tried to see such rare creatures as exemplars of the humanly possible, templates for the generations.
—Kenny Moore

I don't have the stereotypical tall and lean runner's physique. In fact, I sometimes think people look at me and wonder how I've become an elite runner.
—Joan Benoit Samuelson

WES SANTEE

Guys like that never get whipped in their minds. Even when they get beat, they're not beat.

  —Don Humphreys

—◆—

I just don't like to fiddle around. If I was told to get the hoe, I'd run to get it. If I had to go to the barn, I'd run.

  —Wes Santee on his childhood on a ranch

—◆—

Santee's not human.

  —Georgetown coach

—◆—

I didn't think it was so fast.

  —Wes Santee to a reporter after he ran a mile in 4:02.4, an American record

—◆—

Santee struck out above every other athlete like the Aleutian Islands into the Bering Sea.

  —*Des Moines Register*

I don't know when it will be, but I'll run it, you can be sure of that. I'm as certain I can run the four-minute mile as you are that you can drive your car home.
    —Wes Santee to a journalist

———◆———

Santee is the greatest prospect for the four-minute mile America has yet produced. He not only has the physical qualifications, but the mental and spiritual as well.
    —Drake University coach

———◆———

It's like someone pulls you along. I loved to be behind. . . . I judge my pace against his pace, and I'm coming on him. When I catch up and pass, it's great.
    —Wes Santee on competition

FRANK SHORTER

Many people feel that Frank, simply because he won the gold medal in 1972, is inevitably number 1. No matter what I or any other marathoner has done since 1972, Frank is number 1.
    —Bill Rodgers

You're really Frank Shorter, eh? . . . . What happened to you at Montreal?
> —A Charleston cab driver upon learning he was driving Shorter, who
> won Olympic gold in Munich in 1972 and silver in Montreal in 1976.

———◆———

There was something about all those miles, all those minutes of TV coverage through the streets of Munich, something about that silken, light-footed stride and flying hair that lodged forever in our consciousness. Running. Somehow it looked . . . glorious.
> —John Jerome on Shorter's performance at the Munich Marathon in
> 1972

FRANZ STAMPFL

In a way, I knew that he didn't know any better than I did whether or not I would win, because it was a total unknown quantity, but just hearing someone say the things—by then I knew what he would say—was useful.
> —Chris Chataway

———◆———

Fear is the strongest driving-force in competition. Not fear of one's opponent, but of the skill and high standard which he represents; fear, too, of not acquitting oneself well. In the achievement of greater performances, of beating formidable rivals, the athlete defeats fear and conquers himself.
> —Franz Stampfl

He invested with magic this whole painful business of trying to run fast. He made you feel that this would be the most wonderful thing. It would put you along with Michelangelo, Leonardo da Vinci, if you could do it, and he was quite convinced you *could* do it.

—Chris Chataway

PEKKA VASALA

It is suicidal for other runners to copy my hill sessions without adequate background.

—Pekka Vasala, Finnish Middle Distance Runner who outkicked Kip Keino at Munich Olympics in 1972 winning the 1500 meters in 3:36.3

I didn't mind getting second. He's the best in the world.

—Steve Prefontaine

LASSE VIREN

[H]e could win at his will, whenever he decided to go. Everyone just hung around and waited for him to go.

—Frank Shorter

He put his elbows on his knees and just slowly looked around at everyone in the room, one by one, as if to say, "I'm here, guys." And the race was over then. I've never seen a presence like that.

  —Garry Bjorklund on Viren before the 1976 Montreal Olympics

He had a very smooth stride that essentially did not change as he accelerated in the final laps.

  —Frank Shorter

It was like the best chess match you'll ever see. They were outmatched mentally as well as physically.

  —Eino Romppanen on Viren and his opposition at the 1976 Montreal Olympics

[E]verybody has beaten Lasse at one time or another. But nobody beats him at the Olympics.

  —Frank Shorter

In Finland, we have a saying, "Big words don't fell the trees." That's what Lasse did in his running. His races speak louder than his words.

  —Eino Romppanen

Race director Scott Keenan used to say, "Foot races are like horse races; you can either assemble an exciting field, or bring in the Secretariat." That's what Lasse Viren was: a Secretariat.
　　　—Garry Bjorklund

An athlete's career is a brief lightning flash; let me do as much as I can with it before it ends.
　　　—Lasse Viren

Unlike most distance runners, he did not switch to a sprinter's gait in a furious drive to the finish. Somehow he was able to maintain his form . . . and simply run faster.
　　　—Frank Shorter

Lasse was the most talented runner ever.
　　　—Rodolfo Gomez

Sisu is guts, and you know when someone has it. And Lasse had it.
　　　—Eino Romppanen on Viren and the Finnish term *sisu*

PRISCILLA WELCH

Before my marathon in London [in 1981], [Dave] told me I could run three hours, and I ran 2:59. I had to walk near the end, and I was thinking, "Dave said I could do three hours," and so I believed I could.

—Priscilla Welch on her husband

I saw my times improving, and the more I did well, the more I wanted to see what was over the next ridge.

—Priscilla Welch

I was very conscious of how old I was, and that there was so much to do before time ran out. It was like an exciting game.

—Priscilla Welch on becoming a runner

I didn't start out wanting to be an international athlete, but the more I did the better I got.

—Priscilla Welch

Dave saw in Cilla not just the characteristics of a great runner, but also a talent that was far from developed. With a patient, disciplined, but extensive program over time, Dave was able to turn her into one of the foremost marathoners of her time.

—Paul Christman on Dave and Priscilla Welch

I wasn't ever afraid of the cancer, but I was annoyed. It was an interruption, because I was turning 48 and time was getting on for my running. But I heeded the message. And now that I've come out the other end, I can help other ladies go through the same thing.

—Priscilla Welch on her breast cancer

[N]ow I'm focusing on masters, whereas before it was the open. It's getting a lot harder because there's a lot of little jackrabbits in there. The masters division is getting more and more interesting.

—Priscilla Welch

I may want to take up another challenge, use my brains and not my feet. Heaven forbid my brain starts working!

—Priscilla Welch

[I]t's harder to recover from an injury, and it's twice as hard mentally as well.
—Priscilla Welch on getting older

———⊰◆⊱———

You don't even have to run; just do something to keep the body healthy, keep the mind healthy. That way if something does come along, you're able to cope with it.
—Priscilla Welch's advice to breast cancer patients

———⊰◆⊱———

Cilla told me after the race that she reckoned she could take an hour off that time. She didn't realize that if she did, it would be a world record.
—Dave Welch, Priscilla Welch's husband, on Priscilla's first marathon, the Stockholm Marathon, in which she ran a 3:26 and came in ninth

———⊰◆⊱———

Running was exciting, and the more I ran the better I got. It was a fun time, and all so new.
—Priscilla Welch

GRETE WAITZ

If anyone had to choose a queen of the road, it would be Grete Waitz.
—Fred Lebow

Before the race I wasn't nervous. I felt great.

    —Grete Waitz before her first New York City marathon

                  ⟫⟪

The night before the race, we treated ourselves to a nice restaurant complete with a four-course meal of shrimp cocktail, baked potato, red wine, and ice cream.

    —Grete Waitz on the night before her first New York City Marathon, in 1978

                  ⟫⟪

By mile nineteen. . . . I stopped feeling so great. I knew my body had reached unknown territory, never having run so far.

    —Grete Waitz on her first time running the New York City Marathon, in 1978

                  ⟫⟪

My biggest problem was not being able to convert the miles to meters, my measurement system. And since I didn't speak English that well, I was too embarrassed to ask where the heck I was.

    —Grete Waitz

My quads were beginning to cramp so I decided to try and drink water, but I had never experienced this quick form of drinking before and kept spilling the water all over myself. It is definitely an acquired skill, something to be practiced beforehand.

—Grete Waitz

⟹◦⟸

I continued running strong, but having no idea what mile I was on or where this place called Central Park was, I began to get annoyed and frustrated. Every time I saw a patch of trees, I thought, "Oh, this must be Central Park," but no.

—Grete Waitz

EMIL ZATOPEK

Emil is truly the originator of modern intensive training.

—Fred Wilt

⟹◦⟸

Yes, maybe I was not the favorite for 10,000 meters, because there was world-record holder Viljo Heino of Finland. But he was used to practicing near the Arctic Circle, and in London it was a tropical gale, and Heino was unhappy with this climate.

—Emil Zatopek on racing Viljo Heino at the 1948 London Olympics

He thoroughly deserved his success because he is the hardest trained athlete in the world.

—John Landy on Emil Zatopek and his three Olympic gold medals

I understood after the sixth kilometer that I was strong, because [the commentator] says, "After six kilometers, Zatopek is running in better time than Viljo Heino for world record." Oh, really? And the young people yell, "We want world record." And I started to run, and I ran world record.

—Emil Zatopek on a race in 1949

While he goes for a twenty-mile training run on his only free day, we lie here panting with exhaustion, moaning that the gods are unkind to us, and that we're too intelligent to train hard.

—Chris Chataway on Emil Zatopek

Zatopek had no fear of becoming "burned out."

—Fred Wilt

CHAPTER SEVEN

Life lessons in running

"I can't go on, I'll go on"

Although I can be highly competitive when properly self-motivated, sometimes I enter a road race for fun, happy to run with the back of the pack. Of course, all runs are supposed to be fun, but sometimes we lose sight of that fact in our constant desire to run faster, to prove something to ourselves and to others.

I have won four gold medals at the World Masters Championships and five silver and bronze, but sometimes I attend the bi-annual meet merely to signify my presence, not primed to succeed. At the Worlds in Rome one year, after competing on the track and in cross-country, I entered the marathon on the final day mainly as an excuse to run through the streets of the Eternal City, past monuments thousands of years old, without having to worry about being sideswiped by a Fiat. At one point toward the end of the race, I paused on an overlook that offered a view across the Tiber River toward St. Peter's Church. Then I continued to the finish line in the stadium used for the 1960 Olympic Games.

As I crossed the line, an Australian runner finishing in front of me turned and extended his hand, "That's the first time I ever beat you."

Taken by surprise by his comment, fatigued from the week's efforts, I responded with a remark ruder than needed: "You didn't beat me. You merely finished in front of me."

But the words ring true. We should not allow others to define our defeats and victories.

It does not matter how slowly you go so long as you do not stop.
—Confucius

You learn to speak by speaking, to study by studying, to run by running, to work by working; in just the same way, you learn to love by loving.
—Anatole France

Every time I fail I assume I will be a stronger person for it.
—Joan Benoit Samuelson

In our country, our sport is considered something of a miracle. When I won, many discovered that it was finally possible.
—Jelena Prokopcuka, 2005 and 2006 winner of the New York City marathon, on her native Latvia

In general, any form of exercise, if pursued continuously, will help train us in perseverance. Long-distance running is particularly good training in perseverance.
—Mao Tse-Tung

Running is the greatest metaphor for life because you get out of it what you put into it.
  —Oprah Winfrey

——◆——

Life is a marathon, not a sprint; pace yourself accordingly.
  —Amby Burfoot, *The Runner's Guide to the Meaning of Life*

——◆——

I can't go on, I'll go on.
  —Samuel Beckett

——◆——

Executives are like joggers. If you stop a jogger, he goes on running on the spot. If you drag an executive away from his business, he goes on running on the spot, pawing the ground, talking business. He never stops hurtling onwards, making decisions and executing them.
  —Jean Baudrillard, *Cool Memories*

——◆——

Running actually helps with my studies. If I go out and run to the point of depletion and fatigue, all the gunk floating around in my head gets released, so I concentrate better when it's time to hit the books.
  —Ray Steffen

Running has thrown me into adventures that I would otherwise have missed.
—Benjamin Cheever, *Strides*

Sometimes runners think that they can do everything on their own, but support from others is essential, everyone from volunteers and spectators along the course to a helpful spouse who minds the kids while you train.
—Hal Higdon

Running taught me valuable lessons. In cross-country competition, training counted more than intrinsic ability, and I could compensate for a lack of natural aptitude with diligence and discipline. I applied this in everything I did.
—Nelson Mandela

Running in the snow has its own special qualities—softness, quiet, the white landscape—and it can make you feel like a kid again.
—Claire Kowalchik, *The Complete Book of Running for Women*

As a boy, running was always pure joy for me. When I ran I would just let my mind wander and drift. But I would concentrate, too. I would imagine I could fly: *Run harder,* I would tell myself. *I know I can make a life of my own away from this farm.*

　　　　—Haile Gebrselassie, two-time Olympic medalist and holder of the world record for the marathon (2:04:26)

The longer I run, the longer I practice (and I mean that in the meditative sense), the more mysterious the process becomes.

　　　　—Alison Townsend

Farming's a tough life. So is marathoning. Lots of hard work, little time off. Each life conditioned me for the other one.

　　　　—Dick Beardsley

I view life as a series of training events building up to the big race and final finish line and I am always in training, always in the process of reaching the final goal.

　　　　—Matthew Shafner

Maybe people—both able-bodied and amputees—can look at me and say, "You know what? Life is tough, but if this guy can make it, then I can make it."
　　　—Scott Rigsby, who in 2007 became the first double-amputee to complete an Ironman triathlon

Not only in running but in much of life is a sense of balance and proportion necessary.
　　　—Clarence DeMar, 7-time winner of the Boston Marathon

We may outrun
By violent swiftness that which we run at,
And lose by over-running.
　　　—Shakespeare, *Henry VIII*

Each day [running] requires that I inhabit my body as completely as possible, surrender to change, and let that process work on me until I am not the tired and often dispirited woman who leaves the house, but the one who returns enlivened, cheeks aflame, her mind swept clear as a Zen garden.
　　　—Alison Townsend

Success rests in having the courage and endurance and, above all, the will to become the person you are, however peculiar that may be.

—George Sheehan

———◆———

Running is the ultimate tortoise-and-hare activity because the tortoise wins all of the important races. Oh, sure, the hare might get a gold medal at the Olympics or Boston Marathon. But it's the tortoises who continue to run for decades and often even for a lifetime.

—Amby Burfoot, *The Principles of Running*

———◆———

Runners are attuned to their bodies. They sense even tiny physical changes, the kinds that affect performance and general well-being. It was my running that first alerted me to my own illness [cancer], and my running that rehabilitated me from its ravages.

—Fred Lebow

———◆———

My wife says, "You always get your run in". . .Sometimes I wish I devoted more time to my family like a lot of others who are my age, but running has changed my life so much.

—*Bill Rodgers' Lifetime Running Plan*

Pain is inevitable. Suffering is optional.
—Anonymous

If a man coaches himself, then he has only himself to blame when he is beaten.
—Roger Bannister

He ran another hundred yards and he prayed, "Please let me just finish. I don't want to beat anybody. All I want to do is just finish." Because somewhere inside him was the idea that if he could endure it just this one time, then maybe he would get his fair chance, when he could really do something, tomorrow.
—James Buechler, "John Sobieski Burns"

It's not about speed and gold medals. It's about refusing to be stopped.
—Amby Burfoot

In every little village in the world there are great potential champions who only need motivation, development, and good exercise evaluation.
—Arthur Lydiard

Running is a lot like life. Only 10 percent of it is exciting. 90 percent of it is slog and drudge.

> —Dave Bedford, English distance runner who occasionally put in 200 miles a week in training

<hr>

Ask yourself: "Can I give more?" The answer is usually yes.

> —Paul Tergat

<hr>

Pain is temporary, but pride lasts forever.

> —Anonymous

<hr>

Fear is the strongest driving-force in competition. Not fear of one's opponent, but of the skill and high standard which he represents; fear, too, of not acquitting oneself well.

> —Franz Stampfl

<hr>

[A]round a tight bend, take off like holy hell.

> —John Treacy

You can't stop the exterior aging. . . . It's because of health and fitness, and what I eat, and exercise especially, that inside I feel really young.
   —Priscilla Welch

Ignore, then, whether you are tall and thin or short and stocky—whether they laughed at you at home (where they are often unkind) or at school (where they *are* mostly blind, anyway). Indeed—to hell with the lot of them if you "feel" you can do it.
   —Percy Cerutty

It's at the borders of pain and suffering that the men are separated from the boys.
   —Emil Zatopek

Every day you have to test yourself. If you don't, it's a wasted day.
   —Terry Butts, Marine Corps Male Athlete of the Year

Success rests in having the courage and endurance and, above all, the will to become the person you are, however peculiar that may be.
   —George Sheehan

We must all suffer one of two things: the pain of discipline or the pain of regret or disappointment.
  —Jim Rohn

——◆——

Running along a beach at sunrise with no other footprints in the sand, you realize the vastness of creation, your own insignificant space in the plan [. . .] your own creatureliness and how much you owe to the supreme body, the God that brought all this beauty and harmony into being.
  —Sister Marion Irvine

——◆——

[T]he discipline it took to train has entered all facets of my life. I am more focused, get more done during the day.
  —Matthew Shafner

——◆——

As runners, we all go through many transitions—transitions that closely mimic the larger changes we experience in a lifetime. First, we try to run faster. Then we try to run harder. Then we learn to accept ourselves and our limitations, and at last, we can appreciate the true joy and meaning of running.
  —Amby Burfoot

I had to do something to shake up my life and get back some sense of control and trust in the world and along the way fill the hollow space. I needed to rebel against those negative forces, to scream so loud and for so long that the anger living inside me would evacuate forever. But instead of screaming, I ran.

—Gail W. Kislevitz on running after her diagnosis with skin cancer

We went through stages on what to do. My first response was, "Nothing is worth the loss of human life." Then I thought that by stopping the games we'd be doing exactly what the terrorists wanted.

—Frank Shorter on the 1972 Munich Olympics, at which Palestinian terrorists took hostages

I don't believe in striving for extremely fast times and intense levels of competition. I have witnessed the demise of an entire generation of hotshots.

—John Babington, Liberty Athletic Club coach and assistant coach for the 1996 Olympic women's track-and-field team

Once the stopwatch was important for checking splits or a training pace; now I check my watch to pick up the children at school or to meet the babysitter.

—Joan Benoit Samuelson

I have learned that there is no failure in running, or in life, as long as you keep moving.
    —Amby Burfoot

—◦❖◦—

Speed is often confused with insight. When I start running earlier than the others, I appear faster.
    —Johan Cruijff

—◦❖◦—

One chance is all you need.
    —Jesse Owens

—◦❖◦—

Believe in your program, do what you can, be prepared for life's surprises, expect the unexpected.
    —Lorraine Moller on training

—◦❖◦—

There are those of us who are always about to live. We are waiting until things change, until there is more time, until we are less tired, until we get a promotion, until we settle down . . . until, until, until. It always seems as if there is some major event that must occur in our lives before we begin living.
    —George Sheehan

Find the good. It's all around you. Find it, showcase it, and you'll start believing in it.

—Jesse Owens

———◆———

I advise you to say your dream is possible and then overcome all inconveniences, ignore all the hassles and take a running leap through the hoop, even if it is in flames.

—Les Brown

———◆———

Champions are made when no one is watching.

—Anonymous

———◆———

The long run puts the tiger in the cat.

—Bill Squires

———◆———

It's like people always say, "Well, does sport teach you anything in life?" It teaches you certain things, but it doesn't teach you about other things. It doesn't teach, as I say, very much about marriage, very much about how to make a living, any of those things.

—George Plimpton

A runner must run with dreams in his heart, not money in his pocket.
 —Emil Zatopek

———⟫◆⟪———

Know yourself, so you may live that life peculiar to you, the one and only life you were born to live. Know yourself, that you may perfect your body and find your play.
 —George Sheehan

———⟫◆⟪———

You only ever grow as a human being if you're outside your comfort zone.
 —Percy Cerutty

———⟫◆⟪———

I cannot have survival as my only goal. That would be too boring. My goal is to come back in my best running form. It is good for me to have that goal; it will help me.
 —Ludmilla Engquist, Russian-Swedish Olympian who was
  diagnosed with breast cancer in 1999

———⟫◆⟪———

Stadiums are for spectators. We runners have Nature, and that is much better.
 —Juha Vaatainen

You're just running. You're not putting together business plans, solving quadratic equations, or trying to keep your drive from slicing off the fairway.
—Amby Burfoot, *The Runner's Guide to the Meaning of Life*

We never try to put ceilings on anyone. Years ago certain records were unattainable, but it happens. In any given situation in any given time, anything can happen.
—Sue Humphrey

No matter who we are, at some point we are all first-time marathoners. . .We all set goals for ourselves. We all work hard. We all seek to be surrounded by others who will encourage and support us.
—Grete Waitz and Gloria Averbuch, *Run Your First Marathon*

Now if you are going to win any battle you have to do one thing. You have to make the mind run the body. Never let the body tell the mind what to do. The body will always give up. It is always tired morning, noon, and night. But the body is never tired if the mind is not tired. When you were younger the mind could make you dance all night, and the body was never tired. You've always got to make the mind take over and keep going.
—George S. Patton, U.S. Army General and 1912 Olympian

Let him that would move the world first move himself.
　　　—Socrates

———⊰◈⊱———

The most important thing I learned [from running] is that there is only one runner in this race, and that is me.
　　　—George Sheehan

———⊰◈⊱———

Have a dream, make a plan, go for it. You'll get there, I promise.
　　　—Zoe Koplowitz

———⊰◈⊱———

All records fall.
　　　—Amby Burfoot, *The Runner's Guide to the Meaning of Life*

———⊰◈⊱———

It is not necessary for me that you are running. But if you don't run, I'm sure you'll be sorry for it later on.
　　　—Husband of Fanny Blankers-Koen, responding to her request that
　　　　they leave the 1948 Olympics to see their children. She won four
　　　　gold medals at those games.

CHAPTER EIGHT

Motivation and inspiration

"*Just Run*"

As runners we often run alone, climbing out of bed early, donning our shoes and rushing out the door into the darkness of a winter morning to claim our moment of madness before heading to work, what we do when not running. Too little time to call a friend and meet on a corner to break the solitariness of our pursuit. Out of my way, World: Here I come!

Yet other times we crave the company of others. This is one of the main appeals, I am convinced, of the many training programs so popular in large cities, where runners meet to run together to prepare themselves for some major running event, usually a marathon. Certainly this is true with the class offered by the Chicago Area Runners Association, where on a typical weekend morning in the spring and summer several thousand will gather in various locations to prepare for that city's fall marathon.

Thus, sometimes we run as personal entities, and sometimes we gather in groups to bond and share our love of the sport of long distance runner. We can be alone or together. It becomes our personal choice.

You train best where you are the happiest.
  —Frank Shorter

This is what really matters: running. This is where I know where I am.
  —Steve Jones

Tell the truth and run.
  —Yugoslavian proverb

[Y]ou need to start slowly, yes, but you do need to make an effort, you do need to push at times, a little beyond the point of comfort.
  —*Running for Dummies*

Coaches are okay, I guess, but I prefer to do things my own way.
  —Jack Foster

Among the strong, there are the strongest, and behind the able, there are even abler.

    —Chinese proverb

The thinking must be done first, before training begins.

    —Peter Coe

Run when you can, walk if you have to, crawl if you must; just never give up.

    —Dean Karnazes

It is not the doing of it that really counts, but doing it FIRST.

    —Norris McWhirter in *Athletics World*, May 1954

Whether you jog or run is a question of semantics more than commitment or ability.

    —Marc Bloom, *The Runner's Bible*

Fate is never too generous—even to its favorites. Rarely do the gods grant a mortal more than one immortal deed.
    —Stefan Zweig

Generally slow running is considered jogging, but I think you're better off considering yourself a runner from the start.
    —Marc Bloom, *The Runner's Bible*

If you need help getting motivated, turn to fellow runners. Often, they have been there, done that and can help move you along.
    —Hal Higdon

Everybody and their mother knows you don't train hard on Friday, the day before a race. But a lot of runners will over-train on Thursday if left on their own. Thursday is the most dangerous day of the week.
    —Marty Stern, Villanova women's track and cross-country coach

Some people say, "Oh, you're doing only 10-minute miles; you're just a jogger," but it feels like running to me. If you say to yourself you're a runner, you feel more confident, more powerful.
—Kathy Doukas

Fear of trying causes paralysis. Trying causes only trembling and sweating.
—Mason Cooley

Running doesn't have to be monotonous if you put a little imagination into your step.
—Claire Kowalchik, *The Complete Book of Running for Women*

In order to cash in on all the training, get the rest. If you can't run as fast as you want to, you haven't rested enough.
—Ted Corbitt

Remember, the feeling you get from a good run is far better than the feeling you get from sitting around wishing you were running.
—Sarah Condor

You can't flirt with the track. You must marry it.
—Bill Easton

———

There are few instincts more natural than the body in full motion as it races across a field or through the trees.
—Neal Bascomb, *The Perfect Mile*

———

Men's actions are too strong for them. Show me a man who has acted, and who has not been the victim and slave of his action.
—Ralph Waldo Emerson

———

Some days it's not dangerous and some days it is. But I'm staying here to recover and I want to start training again.
—Luke Kibet, marathon gold-medalist at the 2007 World
Championships in Athletics, speaking after being attacked during
the violence that engulfed his native Kenya following the disputed
elections at the end of 2007

———

[M]otivation is a skill. It can be learned and practiced.
—Amby Burfoot

There comes a time late in the afternoon when the light is just so and my circadian rhythms are at exactly a certain point, when the only solid thought in my mind is to *run*.
—Alison Townsend

———◦◦◦———

In the 30 years I've been a runner I've run more than 150,000 miles. Still, some of the hardest steps I take are those first few getting out the door for daily runs.
—*Bill Rodgers' Lifetime Running Plan*

———◦◦◦———

You can't talk yourself into shape. Either you can do it or you can't.
—Frank Shorter

———◦◦◦———

Knowing that I've got a marathon down the road is what gets me to lace up my shoes and head out the door each morning.
—Julie Dworschack

———◦◦◦———

My coworkers and non-running friends, even my husband, tend to think I am weird for running. I get tired of defending myself, of trying to make them understand what it means to me. With my running friends, I don't have to go through all that.
—Kim Ahrens

I trotted on along the edge of a field bordered by the sunken lane, smelling green grass and honeysuckle, and I felt as though I came from a long line of whippets trained to run on two legs.

— Alan Sillitoe, "The Loneliness of the Long-Distance Runner"

———✦———

I don't believe in burnout. I believe in losing your appetite.

— Pat Tyson

———✦———

Your shoes are only as good as the laces they're attached to.

— Greg Sampson

———✦———

Some people endure pain better than others. All things considered, the ability to withstand—or even deny—pain would seem to be a valuable ally for the long distance runner in search of significant improvement. In truth, it is probably a double-edged sword, since medical experts tell us that pain is the body's warning signal to back off, and that to ignore such schedules is to roll the dice with both body and mind.

— Mark Will-Weber

Top results are reached only through pain. But eventually you like this pain. You'll find the more difficulties you have on the way, the more you will enjoy your success.
    —Juha "The Cruel" Väätäinen

⬥

Nothing's better than the wind to your back, the sun in front of you, and your friends beside you.
    —Aaron Douglas Trimble

⬥

Those who say that I will lose and am finished will have to run over my body to beat me.
    —Said Aouita

⬥

Running with others can help get you out when you might otherwise blow it off.
    —Frank Shorter

⬥

Avoid running at all times.
    —Satchel Paige

[R]unning is a year-round sport and you train for all conditions, so you sort of have to be mentally prepared, physically sort of used to it.
     —Bill Rodgers

⊷◆⊶

But if you can find that spot—I suppose it's like running—I used to be a swimmer and swim laps, and you just have to be there with what you're doing.
     —Bruce Nauman

⊷◆⊶

I have my routine. I'm running three or four miles a day.
     —Dirk Benedict

⊷◆⊶

To keep motivated, I started swearing at my husband for getting me into this mess in the first place.
     —Grete Waitz on her first time running the New York City
        Marathon, in 1978

⊷◆⊶

I believe 100 percent in continued running after forty, and racing too, if one so desires.
     —Bill Rodgers

How can one learn to know oneself? Never by introspection, rather by action.
—Johann Wolfgang Von Goethe

———◆———

When I was young, I was too slow. I thought I must learn to run fast by practicing to run fast, so I ran 100 meters fast 20 times. Then I came back slow, slow, slow. People said, "Emil, you are crazy. You are training like a sprinter."
—Emil Zatopek

———◆———

Somewhere in the world someone is training when you are not. When you race him, he will win.
—Tom Fleming's Boston Marathon Training Motto

———◆———

Runners like to train 100 miles per week because it's a round number. But I think 88 is a lot rounder.
—Don Kardong

———◆———

There's no such thing as bad weather, just soft people.
—Bill Bowerman

If one can stick to the training throughout the many long years, then will power is no longer a problem. It's raining? That doesn't matter. I am tired? That's besides the point. It's simply that I just have to.

  —Emil Zatopek

Sometimes . . . an injury may be due to increased running, fatigue, sickness, etc. and have nothing at all to do with your shoe.

  —Bill Rodgers

He that would be a great man must learn to turn every accident to some advantage.

  —Francois Duc de la Rochefoucauld

Experience has taught me how important it is to just keep going, focusing on running fast and relaxed. Eventually [pain] passes and the flow returns. It's part of racing.

  —Frank Shorter

When a person trains once, nothing happens. When a person forces himself to do a thing a hundred or a thousand times, then he certainly has developed in more ways than physical.

 —Emil Zatopek

During the hard training phase, never be afraid to take a day off. If your legs are feeling unduly stiff and sore, rest; if you are at all sluggish, rest; in fact, if in doubt, rest.

 —Bruce Fordyce

If you train hard, you'll not only be hard, you'll be hard to beat.

 —Herschel Walker

Train, don't strain.

 —Arthur Lydiard

There are twenty ways of going to a point, and one is the shortest; but set out at once on one.

 —Ralph Waldo Emerson

I tell the kids to have "wide eyes," to run light as a feather, to get high on their toes, and to dig deep, dig deep, dig deep!
  —Pat Tyson

———◆———

Let your running lead you to your diet.
  —Bill Rodgers

———◆———

No amount of junk miles, fun runs or affirmations are going to get you over the hill at the five-mile mark in a 10k. However, what will pull you through is solid prep with hard hill runs and interval work.
  —Manciata

———◆———

Dwell on the positive, but have controlled, passionate anger.
  —Pat Tyson

———◆———

Run hard, be strong, think big!
  —Percy Cerutty

I believe in keeping running simple and, in regard to shoes, that would mean no gimmicks, unnecessary cushioning, etc.
　　—Bill Rodgers

———◆———

Don't attack a hill from the very bottom—it's bigger than you are!
　　—Harry Groves, Penn State coach

———◆———

See what you are about to do as a thing that has already been accomplished; it will in fact help you do it. The race will already be run before you run it.
　　—*The Runner's Book of Daily Inspiration*, Kevin Nelson

———◆———

You would fain be victor at the Olympic games, you say. Yes, but weigh the conditions, weigh the consequences; then and then only, lay to your hand if it be for your profit.
　　—Epictetus

———◆———

Physiologists and high-performance trainers understand now that the concept of 110 percent is no longer a smart way to train. Give 110 percent, and you won't build your body up, but actually break it down. And be no good to yourself or anyone else.
　　—Sally Jenkins, the *Washington Post*

Thus I urge you to go on to your greatness if you believe it is in you. Think deeply and separate what you wish from what you are prepared to do.
— Percy Cerutty

⟫—⟪

The more I talk to athletes, the more convinced I become that the method of training is relatively unimportant. There are many ways to the top, and the training method you choose is just the one that suits you best. No, the important thing is the attitude of the athlete, the desire to get to the top.
— Herb Elliott

⟫—⟪

Even during the height of the war in neighboring Bosnia, Dejan Nikolic persisted in putting on the Belgrade Marathon. . . . [D]espite the difficulties, Nikolic insisted that the marathon must continue because, he said, he wanted "to show the world that runners have so much in common."
— Michael Sandrock

⟫—⟪

If the coach cannot do it, he cannot "teach" it—only talk about it.
— Percy Cerutty

The Zulu warrior women could run fifty miles a day and fight at the end of it. Fifty miles together, perfectly in step, so the veldt drummed with it. Did their hearts beat as one? My heart can beat with theirs, slow and strong and efficient— pumping energy.

—Sara Maitland, "The Loveliness of the Long-Distance Runner"

Even a runner who is running alone has friends among the squirrels, rocks, snowy egrets, pines, eucalyptus, and wild hay.

—Kevin Nelson, *The Runner's Book of Daily Inspiration*

[F]or me, like so many others, running is the answer. Out on the road it is just you, the pavement, and your will.

—John Bingham, *The Courage to Start*

He began to run. Almost immediately he felt easier; felt confidence flow through him as though it were his blood; felt that now, at last, he was in his own country or, more accurately, in his own medium.

—Harry Sylvester, "Going to Run All Night"

Don't bother just to be better than your contemporaries or predecessors. Try to be better than yourself.
—William Faulkner

———⊷———

It's not about how fast you go. It's not about how far you go. It's a process.
—Amby Burfoot, *The Runner's Guide to the Meaning of Life*

———⊷———

Running is my meditation, mind flush, cosmic telephone, mood elevator, and spiritual communion.
—Lorraine Moller

CHAPTER NINE

Why runners run

Runner's High

A discussion among participants on my Internet bulletin boards suggested that many of those responding claimed to have experienced the mythical "Runner's High." Others had not. Among the others, I suspect that it was less that they had not experienced the High, but more that they simply failed to recognize it.

Is the High some gargantuan "When Harry Met Sally" orgasm, or is it simply a general feeling of well being we feel now and then when we run?

Scientists have attempted to explain the Runner's High by suggesting that exercise releases endorphins into the brain triggering the emotion, but the evidence seems scanty. I seek less scientific explanations:

If you head down the road without proper warm-up, it may take 10 or 15 minutes to get up to speed in an hour-long run. Then another 10 or 15 minutes to work out all the kinks in your stride so that you are moving smoothly, breathing right. Because you have not yet run far enough to experience extreme fatigue, you start feeling good. And for that third period encompassing 10 or 15 minutes, you encounter what author John Jerome referred to in a book as the "Sweet Spot in Time." Whether at a High or not, you are capable of moving as fast as you can while expending seemingly small amounts of energy. Then fatigue grabs you by the throat, forcing a slowdown during the last 10 or 15 minutes. If you time it right and don't push too hard at the end, you should finish refreshed, feeling a sense of great accomplishment.

Is this the elusive Runner's High? I don't know, but seeking this Sweet Spot is one reason I keep running. I have many reasons. And so does everyone else.

I believe in the runner's high, and I believe that those who are passionate about running are the ones who experience it to the fullest degree possible

—Sasha Azevedo

The true but rare runner's high is a zone that we enter when everything seems to click perfectly, when time stands still, and when we can run almost without effort.

—Amby Burfoot, *The Runner's Guide to the Meaning of Life*

Adrenaline dispels boredom. Run, you sufferers from ennui! Run for your lives!

—Mason Cooley, *City Aphorisms*

Running improves my relationships with my family, my friends, everyone around me. And while my running is personal, it's also something I give. Running can be given.

—Tony Sandoval, M.D., winner of the 1980 U.S. Olympic Marathon Trials

---

Running became the one event in my daily life that I looked forward to. Books and movies paled in comparison to the refuge of my feet slapping patiently in the fresh morning air.

—Kate Kinsey

He seems to run from within himself.
>   —Emil Zatopek on Haile Gebrselassie

I still bother with runners I call hamburgers. They're never going to run any record times. But they can fulfill their own potential.
>   —Bill Bowerman

Life is short. Running makes it seem longer.
>   —Baron Hansen

Running was the time he felt most alive. He knew that as surely as he'd ever known anything.
>   —Richard Christian Matheson, "Third Wind"

Fitness is a stage you pass through on the way to becoming a runner.
>   —George Sheehan

Running helps me stay on an even keel and in an optimistic frame of mind.
　　—Bill Clinton

My eyes burned with sweat, and I squinted so tight I could hardly see anymore, and because they stung it was impossible to think. I was adjusting, though, lost in rhythm, like a mechanical animal caught on the rim of existence . . . it felt good and I was slipping deep in dreams.
　　—Walter McDonald, "The Track"

It's just simply that I have to.
　　—Emil Zatopek

Running is a great way to relieve stress and clear the mind.
　　—Joan Van Ark

My suspicion is that the effects of running are not extraordinary at all, but quite ordinary. It is the other states, all other feelings, that are peculiar, for they are an abnegation of the way you and I are supposed to feel. As runners, I think we reach directly back along the endless chain of history.
　　—James W. Fixx, *The Complete Book of Running*

Sometimes I'll have a problem while working on a piece and I'll say, "Wait a second, I need a break." I get our spaniel, Thunder, head out for a run, and 50 minutes later, when I try the passage again, it's easy. Running clears the head.

—Misha Dichter, classical pianist

⟫◆⟪

I am not sure that I can describe what has been called the "runner's high," but like poetry and beauty, I know it when I experience it.

—Matthew Shafner

⟫◆⟪

My feelings tried to control me on my run. I had to concentrate fully on forthcoming running and success. I wanted to triumph.

—Cathy Freeman

⟫◆⟪

You have to wonder at times what you're doing out there. Over the years, I've given myself a thousand reasons to keep running, but it always comes back to where it started. It comes down to self-satisfaction and a sense of achievement.

—Steve Prefontaine

⟫◆⟪

I can't imagine living and not running.

—Paula Radcliffe

It is the athlete's job to learn to do the hard things easily.
 —John Jerome, *The Sweet Spot in Time*

My times become slower and slower, but the experience of the race is unchanged: each race a drama, each race a challenge, each race stretching me in one way or another, and each race telling me more about myself and others.
 —George Sheehan

I do a lot of running and hiking, and I also collect stamps.
 —Sally Ride

I always have loved running, since I was fifteen.
 —Bill Rodgers

I loved the feeling of freedom in running, the fresh air, the feeling that the only person I'm competing with is me.
 —Wilma Rudolph

I enjoy the freedom of running and the challenge of training and competition as much now as when I first started back in high school.

—Alberto Salazar

———⋗•⋖———

For me, running is a lifestyle and an art. I'm more interested in the magic of it than the mechanics.

—Lorraine Moller

———⋗•⋖———

My running was very simple; it was out of myself. Perhaps sometimes I was like a mad dog. It didn't matter about style or what it looked like to others; there were records to break.

—Emil Zatopek

———⋗•⋖———

To me, the runner's high is a sensational reaction to a great run! It's an exhilarating feeling of satisfaction and achievement.

—Sasha Azevedo

I read somewhere that when you run for longer than an hour, your body begins to adapt in miraculous ways. I couldn't actually have thought, even then, that my arteries were growing, but it was like that. I'd go for a 20 and glance down at my sternum, like a hen sitting on an egg.

—Benjamin Cheever, *Strides*

<hr/>

Mr. Rodgers, why don't you concentrate more on your vocation rather than your avocation.

—the school principal, to Bill Rodgers, at the school where Rodgers taught for a living

<hr/>

I always loved running . . . it was something you could do by yourself, and under your own power. You could go in any direction, fast or slow as you wanted, fighting the wind if you felt like it, seeking out new sights just on the strength of your feet and the courage of your lungs.

—Jesse Owens

<hr/>

If one could run without getting tired, I don't think one would often want to do anything else.

—C.S. Lewis

I feel the earth and the wind and the trees. I feel its spirit. It puts me in the moment. I feel the rhythm of the race. It's like music. When the rhythm gets dissonant and chaotic, it is either a jazzy driving force behind me or demons inside me.

—Gabriel Jennings

Everyone wants beautiful legs.

—Peter Martins and New York City Ballet, *New York City Ballet Workout*

There is no such thing as an average runner. We are all above average.

—Hal Higdon, *Marathoning A to Z*

I didn't want to run Boston to prove anything. I just fell in love with the marathon.

—Roberta Gibb on running the Boston Marathon

I like running because it's a challenge. If you run hard, there's the pain—and you've got to work your way through the pain. You know, lately it seems all you hear is "Don't overdo it" and "Don't push yourself." Well, I think that's a lot of bull. If you push the human body, it will respond.

    —Bob Clarke, Philadelphia Flyers general manager, NHL Hall of Fame

CHAPTER TEN

Witty running commentary

A Funny Thing Happened on the Way to the Finish Line

We runners are a motley bunch. Consider how we dress, specifically before a marathon. Given our high demographics, we should look like bankers and fashion models wearing Pradas and Brooks Brothers suits, but we arrive at the Expo one notch above the Homeless.

Muddied running shoes. Faded jeans. Aged T-shirt from one race. Billed cap from another. Nylon jacket from a third. The highest fashion statement we can make is that we acquired that jacket at the Boston Marathon, 100th running in 1996, meaning it has been thrown in the washer one hundred times.

But we are the chosen people, who arrive at the starting line dressed in upside-down garbage bags carrying bottles with yellowed liquid: Gatorade before we drink, urine afterwards. During the course of our 26-mile-385-yard journeys, we acquire: a) bloody nipples, b) black toes and c) so much salt clinging to our bodies that it appears we just took a swim in the Dead Sea.

And as we stagger through the streets, spectators shout from the sidelines, "You're looking good!"

Once finished, we collapse into the arms of some stranger who wraps around our sunburned shoulders a Mylar blanket that crinkles as we walk and displays the name of some bank, shoe company or department store. We have just paid $100 to enter this race, and now we have to spend the rest of the day looking like an aluminum billboard. And even if we have not barfed up that Gatorade, you do not want to kiss us.

The next day, however, we do look good: with that finisher's medal hung around our shoulders.

Running is like mouthwash; if you can feel the burn, it's working.
　　—Brian Tackett

———⊰◈⊱———

My most vivid memories of beginning to run are of how little anyone seemed to know about the sport and how little was available in way of information and equipment. . .when I went to a newsstand to try to find a running magazine, it was hopeless. "Running," I told the vendor, who looked quite puzzled. "You know—track and field." His eyes lit up in seeming recognition. Then he handed me *Road & Track*, a magazine about cars.
　　—Fred Lebow

———⊰◈⊱———

I'll get up in the morning while they've all got hangovers and run my five miles. But the women who do run are usually ten years younger than me and they're really obsessed about running. That's all they do. They're really boring.
　　—Trisha Goddard

Before he rounds the brushy curves, we see him, his French running shoes, his shorts, his naked legs, his T-shirt advertising something unimaginable, his terry sweatband, his tiny nylon wallet fastened to his shoe ingeniously with Velcro—who once was never seen without a coat and necktie—hairy wool, rumpled linen, bleached-to-the-bone starched cotton broadcloth, stained shimmering reptilian silk—who hated zippers as much as polyester, snaps as much as leisure suits.

    —Lon Otto, "We Cannot Save Him"

The pleasure of jogging and running is rather like that of wearing a fur coat in Texas in August: the true joy comes in being able to take the damn thing off.

    —Joseph Epstein

If you come to think of it, you never see deer, dogs, and rabbits worrying about their menus, and yet they run much faster than humans.

    —Emil Zatopek

Even in high school, you were some kind of fruitcake if you ran, like you were naked in the wind. Nobody else did it; there were no cheerleaders or anything like that.

    —Charlie Rodgers

Lady, you just passed it.

    —Spectator to Joan Benoit Samuelson, when she asked in the 1979
    Boston Marathon how far away Heartbreak Hill was

<hr>

Dick Cheney said he was running again. He said his health was fine. "I've got a doctor with me twenty-four hours a day." Yeah, that's always the sign of a man in good health, isn't it?

    —David Letterman

<hr>

Runner's high? Isn't that where two runners pass in the park and one says, "Hi." And the other returns the greeting?

    —Hal Higdon

<hr>

I signed up for track in high school as it was the easiest team to join; no cuts and everyone is guaranteed a position.

    —Kim Ahrens

<hr>

Sweat cleanses from the inside. It comes from places a shower will never reach.

    —George Sheehan

I've never seen a computer jogging.
> —Basketball coach Frank Layden on why computers are smarter than
> people

Hell, no. When I die I want to be sick.
> —Abe Lemons when asked if he runs

I guess the difference is that running makes me feel good, and the other stuff
makes me feel bad.
> —Don Imus on being addicted to running versus being addicted to
> smoking and drinking

I learned not to take the lead if I wasn't sure where the finish line was.
> —Pat Petersen, who got lost in his first high-school cross country race

---

After the first six-mile loop, Harry Murphy . . . offered me a cup of whisky. I
gulped it down . . . After the next six-mile loop, I happily downed another cup of
whisky. On the third loop, someone gave me a cup of water. I was so disappointed!
> —Fred Lebow on his experience at the Cherry Tree Marathon in the
> Bronx in 1970

"A sunny day in winter" is a nice way of describing the seasoned runner. I've heard worse.
  —Roger Robinson

❖

When I jog I joggle.
  —Ogden Nash

❖

Two things are bad for the heart—running uphill and running down people.
  —Bernard Gimbel

❖

I am quite sure she was under the impression that I had run four miles in one minute.
   —Roger Bannister on his girlfriend Moyra Jacobsson's lack of interest in his running

❖

Distance-running, to a professional athlete in my day, was five laps around the field. And you stopped each lap to take your pulse.
  —Lynn Swann

While running, it is rude to count the people you pass out loud.
—Anonymous

———◆———

Even if you fall flat on your face at least you are moving forward.
—Sue Luke

———◆———

Maybe I shouldn't have had breakfast at Denny's.
—Jordan Kent, who vomited after running the 400 meters in the 2002 USA Junior National Championships held in Eugene, OR

———◆———

Running on worn-out shoes is like driving on bald tires. You might make the next town, but then again, you might have a blow out.
—Running shop owner

———◆———

In the very first race in literature, the old guy wins. He's Odysseus (AKA Ulysses), pushing forty at the time, and he beats the best of the united Greek army gathered outside Troy.
—Roger Robinson

[R]unning in a pretty muddy cross country race, one of my shoes stuck in the mud and came off. . . . I really got aggressive with myself, and [started] to pass a lot of runners. . . . I improved something like twenty places. . . . But I never did get my shoe back.
—Rob de Castella

If you grunt, grimace, grind, and pound your way through a run and then you limp home 15 minutes later, you may want to consider changing your style.
—*Running for Dummies*

Kids can watch [other sports] start to finish, in real time. . . . But the men's 400 relay finals at the world championships? On your mark, get set . . . we'll show it to you in four hours on another network.
—Mike Penner, "Track and Field, TV Has a Problem with You," Los *Angeles Times*, August 13, 2001

I said running a sub-2:20 would be a cakewalk after this.
—Joan Benoit Samuelson on giving birth to her daughter

A critic is a legless man who teaches running.
    —Channing Pollock

———⟶◆⟵———

If the hill has its own name, then it's probably a pretty tough hill.
    —Marty Stern

———⟶◆⟵———

Only one hill today, boys.
    —Jock Semple, at the start of the Mount Washington Road Race

———⟶◆⟵———

The first time I see a jogger smiling, I'll consider it.
    —Joan Rivers

———⟶◆⟵———

Have you ever noticed? Anyone going slower than you is an idiot, and anyone going faster than you is a maniac?
    —George Carlin

I will even try eating worms and caterpillar fungus. It might improve my jogging, and for sure it will improve my flossing.
—Scott Ostler in the *San Francisco Chronicle*

———⟫✦⟪———

There ain't no shame looking at a good runner's back. Now, if the runner sucks, that's something else entirely. . .
—The Rage, Training Tips, "Comeback"

———⟫✦⟪———

The event that certainly tries men's soles.
—Jerry Nason on the Boston Marathon, in 1945

———⟫✦⟪———

If you are noticing the scenery, you probably aren't working hard.
—Sebastian Coe

———⟫✦⟪———

If you run every day until you're 90 years old, I guarantee that you'll live a long life.
—*Bill Rodgers' Lifetime Running Plan*

There are actually people who cheat at race walks.... You know you've given up in life when you cheat at a race walk. You've decided that you're so pathetic the only way you can win is by cheating against people who aren't even competing.
  —Michael Logsdon

       ⋙—◆—⋘

If you ask my younger daughter what I do, she'll tell you that I'm the fastest runner in the world. In other words, she doesn't know much about running.
  —*Bill Rodgers' Lifetime Running Plan*

       ⋙—◆—⋘

If you want to know what you'll look like in ten years, look in the mirror after you've run a marathon.
  —Jeff Scaff

       ⋙—◆—⋘

Hills: You entered a marathon with hills? You idiot.
  —Don Kardong's marathon advice

       ⋙—◆—⋘

Who runs in circles never gets far.
  —Thornton W. Burgess, Bowser the Hound

Running won't kill you, you'll pass out first!
—Anonymous

[W]hen I go to competitions the young girls don't look upon me as a granny. Except if you are Uta Pippig. One day I was out training, and she said to me, "Heh, Cilla, you could be my mother."
—Priscilla Welch

I go running when I have to. When the ice cream truck is doing sixty.
—Wendy Liebman

To a runner, a side stitch is like a car alarm. It signifies something is wrong, but you ignore it until it goes away.
—Anonymous

It's unnatural for people to run around the city streets unless they are thieves or victims. It makes people nervous to see someone running. I know that when I see someone running on my street, my instincts tell me to let the dog go after him.
—Mike Royko

I don't generally like running. I believe in training by rising gently up and down from the bench.

> —Satchel Paige

School cross country runs started because the rugby pitches were flooded. There was an alternative: extra studying. This meant there were plenty of runners on sports afternoons.

> —Gordon Pirie

I believe that the Good Lord gave us a finite number of heartbeats and I'm damned if I'm going to use up mine running up and down a street.

> —Neil Armstrong

I don't think jogging is healthy, especially morning jogging. If morning joggers knew how tempting they looked to morning motorists, they would stay home and do sit-ups.

> —Rita Rudner

Runners just do it—they run for the finish line even if someone else has reached it first.

  —Anonymous

"Why aren't you signed up for the 401K?"
"I'd never be able to run that far."
  —Scott Adams, *Dilbert* (4/2/01)

I get my exercise running to the funerals of my friends who exercise.
  —Barry Gray

Technically, these guys did not run entirely from coast to coast contiguously, because they crossed the Hudson River and Mississippi River by ferry.
  —Paul Reese, Cross USA runner, who covered both rivers by running across bridges, speaking of earlier runners.

Most of the top runners I know feel the same way about diet. They're skeptical about nutrition being the prime element in racing success, but they like to check each other's grocery lists. Just in case.
  —Don Kardong

I am not ashamed to say that I don't like to *run* anywhere, unless it's really extremely urgent, like if I pull into the Denny's parking lot at 4:59, knowing the Senior Dinner Discount stops at 5:00. Also, I've recently discovered that when I run anywhere at my age, my belly button arrives at my destination about three minutes before I do.
 —Michael Milligan, *Grandpa Rules*

———◆———

Practice doesn't make perfect. Perfect practice makes perfect.
 —Peter Martins and New York City Ballet, *New York City Ballet Workout*

———◆———

Running is the best anti-depressant on the market, with virtually no cost or negative side effects.
 —Hal Higdon, *Marathoning A to Z*

CHAPTER ELEVEN

Our "Gigantic" running miscellany

Running with the Pack, Part II

Is there a lovelier piece of music than Mozart's 21st piano concerto, the C-Major? The second movement served as the theme song for the 1967 Swedish film, *Elvira Madigan*, but most of those running marathons today were not even born before that year. They train wearing iPods tuned to electronic beats, not subtle melodies written by some eighteenth century composer.

I don't own an iPod, and despite my love of Mozart, I concede that his 21st piano concerto would be a poor choice for working out. You'd get off to a good start with the first movement, the *Allegro* (or fast), but then you collide with the second movement, marked *Andante*, a word that tells the orchestra to play it slowly. It would bring you to a halt as a runner. Even the tumultuous Rondo in the third and final movement, another *Allegro*, might not get you moving again.

Nevertheless, the waters of classical music run deep, not shallow. As runners, we can learn as much from the format in which the music is written as from the music itself. When I write training programs for runners, I usually prescribe a hard day to push the muscles, followed by an easy day to rest them, followed by another hard day to build on what went before. *Allegro, Andante, Allegro.* Oregon coach Bill Bowerman pioneered the hard/easy approach.

Mozart knew how to blend fast and slow movements just as Bowerman knew how to blend fast and slow workouts.

It may be a stretch to suggest that Mozart can teach us how to train for road races. Maybe it is enough merely to enjoy his music, still popular today even on some iPods, then run to your own beat.

I have to train him not only to represent Michigan. I have to train him to represent the United States.
  —Ron Warhurst on Alan Webb

——◆——

Every time I have a personal or work problem, I go for a run.
  —Fred Lebow

——◆——

Every day is a good day when you run.
  —Kevin Nelson, *The Runner's Book of Daily Inspiration*

——◆——

You start pounding out a couple dozen 5- or 6-minute miles and you start to feel such a sense of satisfaction and peace you can't believe it. Sure you're tired, and sure you're sore, but if you could bottle the high you get from transcending the pain mile after mile after mile, well . . . reality was overrated.
  —Dick Beardsley

——◆——

Running made us human, at least in an anatomical sense.
  —Dr. Daniel E. Lieberman

It was a carnival of pain, but he loved each stride because the running distilled him to essence and the heat hastened this distillation.
—James Tabor, "The Runner"

I don't know when I made the transformation from running as a sport to running as part of my life. I can't separate the two.
—Gail W. Kislevitz

We are here to be heroes. The marathon is the one way we prove it to ourselves.
—George Sheehan

At twenty miles I wanted to cry. . . . I needed nourishment in the worst way and then I spotted a Dairy Queen across the street. Soft ice cream, the perfect food!
—Richard Bellicchi

There is something about running that knocks down the "Berlin Walls" of race, religion, custom, and language that divide us, reminding us—as Alberto Juantorena says—that we all have "not four eyes, but two."
—Michael Sandrock

I didn't just want to run, I wanted to run as far and as fast as I could, as was humanly possible.
　　—Ted Corbitt

———◆◆◆———

I read in the sports section about Roger Bannister breaking the four-minute mile. I couldn't comprehend the speed of a four-minute mile, so I got on my bike, rode to Wingate Field which had a track, climbed over the three-tier cyclone fence, and ran around the track once as fast as I could and timed myself at 1:25.
　　—Nina Kuscsik

———◆◆◆———

I do think there are lots of kids out there who have the potential to be great runners if only they have the right coach, someone who shows an interest and cares.
　　—Bill Rodgers

———◆◆◆———

When I took my artificial right leg for a 26.2-mile run in 1976, I had no idea how it would change my life. I entered the New York City Marathon that year because I was a runner and that is what runners do.
　　—Dick Traum

I never was a good track runner; psychologically, the laps killed me.
—Kathrine Switzer

———◆———

This is not about instant gratification. You have to work hard for it, sweat for it, give up sleeping in on Sunday mornings.
—Lauren Fessenden

———◆———

The input is considerable but the rewards are unbelievable.
—Rob Hemmel

———◆———

Running changed my life and brought it into balance. I now feel as though my entire essence, body, and soul is centered.
—Donna Isaacson

———◆———

There's nothing quite like your first marathon. The adrenaline just flows.
—Sister Marion Irvine

It didn't matter that we were last. We knew we were finishing, that we would endure to the end.
—Thomas King

I died at twenty miles. I was tired and thought, I will never do this again. This is crazy. Even Kenyans get tired after running that far.
—Paul Mbugua

Stopping is an honorable tradition in running.
—Kevin Nelson, *The Runner's Book of Daily Inspiration*

This was definitely harder than any track course I had run. . . . I didn't like this marathon racing.
—Grete Waitz on her first marathon

It was a whole different game once we got to the hills. We had been running really slow, and from my point of view that was fine. But once we started up, he began pushing the pace at an intensity that neither of us could continue to the finish. It was only a matter of time before either he would break me, or he would have to slow down himself.

> —Alberto Salazar on the competition between him and Dick Beardsley at the 1982 Boston Marathon

———◆———

[W]omen like Olympian Paula Radcliffe have world record marathon times that are sub-2:20—that's more than two hours faster than the first woman known to run a marathon in 1896.

> —Shanti Sosienski, *Women Who Run*

———◆———

Nothing hurts more, but is so rewarding at the same time.

> —Sandy Zanchi on the marathon

———◆———

What if this were your only chance? Sure, it'll be painful, but what's pain?

> —Franz Stampfl

Do you not know that in a race all the runners run, but only one gets the prize. Run in such a way as to get the prize.
    —St. Paul, Corinthians 9:24

We all need goals. Life is hard to live without one.
    —Tory Baucum

[Running] pervades my life. I wouldn't go so far as to say it has crept into other parts of my life; I would rather say it has become its own part of my life.
    —Larry Smith

[Running] is my private time, my therapy, my religion.
    —Gail W. Kislevitz

The combined feeling of exhaustion, euphoria, and accomplishment is quite luxurious.
    —Larry Smith on how it feels after finishing a marathon

On a good day, it all blends. I feel a part of a private universe where everything comes together and feels great.
  —Matthew Shafner

⧓

I had to learn how to drink while running. That sounds easy, but it's like rubbing your head and patting your stomach at the same time.
  —Kim Ahrens

⧓

I couldn't fail, as no other amputee had ever attempted to run a marathon before.
  —Dick Traum

⧓

I definitely think the high school coaches should take the opportunity to educate runners that this is a sport that will take them through life.
  —Kim Ahrens

⧓

That was the first time I had seen runners at close quarters. They appeared as normal human beings, not demigods as I had imagined.
  —Kenyan runner Paul Tergat on seeing runners at the All-African
   games as a child

Pasta (despite some recent attacks that question just how much nutritional punch the noodle wields) has traditionally been the darling of the pre-race meal.
    —Mark Will-Weber

⟹•⟸

He took in even, deep measures of cool air with mechanical regularity, disinterestedly feeling inside his chest the huge heart muscle thumping its slow liquid drumbeat.
    —John L. Parker Jr., *Once a Runner*

⟹•⟸

[A]t age forty-three, when I found myself standing in my garage in a new pair of running shoes, I knew that it was my moment of truth . . . Behind me lay forty years of bad decisions and broken promises.
    —John Bingham, *The Courage to Start*

⟹•⟸

Running is a kind of investment in yourself.
    —*The Runner's Book of Daily Inspiration*, Kevin Nelson

⟹•⟸

It has been said that the love of the chase is an inherent delight in man—a relic of an instinctive passion.
    —Charles Darwin

The fastest human can run about 10 meters a second for about 10 seconds. Your typical squirrel can double that for 4 or 5 minutes.

—Dr. Daniel E. Lieberman

———◆◆◇———

Today, [endurance running] is primarily a form of exercise and recreation, but its roots may be as ancient as the origin of the human genus, and its demands a major contributing factor to the human body form.

—*Nature*

———◆◆◇———

When we understand the privilege of what it means to be an athlete, we are in touch with, and rejoice in, our physical, mental, and emotional strengths and our endless possibilities.

—Gloria Averbuch

———◆◆◇———

He felt good. Loose, with lots of juice in his flat-muscled body and an easy animal grace that brought the road back under him in long effortless strides.

—George Harmon Coxe, "See How They Run"

———◆◆◇———

Although he was not a very good runner, he knew all about running.

—Harry Sylvester, "Going to Run All Night"

Consistency requires discipline. Force yourself out the door.
—Bob Glover and Shelly-Lynn Florence Glover, *The Competitive Runner's Handbook*

—◆—

When he hears the gun, his muscles will automatically spring to action. He can almost feel the breeze that will flow smoothly over his face and arms and legs. His spikes will rhythmically splash cinder behind him and there will be cheering from the bleachers to his right.
—Louis Edwards, "Ten Seconds"

—◆—

The feel of that day was still in his limbs: he remembered the vague glow of promise, the sense of being released as he sped over the turf of roughly prepared track—effortless, as though his body had lightened, brought to a pitch of harmony by the simple miracle of the up-drawing sun.
—George Ewart Evans, "The Medal"

—◆—

I don't consider hard work and great fun mutually exclusive. Who decided that anyway?
—Dick Beardsley

Experienced runners learn to respect the changing needs of their bodies. That's the wisdom that comes with time, and—for good or bad—with age.

 —Fred Lebow

——◆——

At first an ordeal and then an accomplishment, the daily run becomes a staple, like bread, or wine, a fine marriage, or air. It is also a free pass to friendship.

 —Benjamin Cheever, *Strides*

——◆——

Out of a silver heat mirage he ran. Two lanes of blacktop stretched straight and flat in front of him, straight and flat behind. August-tall corn walled in the road and its red-sand shoulders. A half mile away was a blue-dark wall of woods.

 —James Tabor, "The Runner"

——◆——

Running was the time he felt most alive. He knew that as surely as he'd ever known anything.

 —Richard Christian Matheson, "Third Wind"

I waited for someone to speak, but all ran quietly, all alone. Now and then we would fall into step and there would be the thump thump thump of our running. Then the steps would syncopate and break rhythm and in the heavy depressing heat I would find myself having to concentrate to maintain stride.

—Walter McDonald, "The Track"

———⟫•⟪———

I couldn't admit this for many years, but I was afraid that if I took a break from running I'd lose it.

—Dick Beardsley

———⟫•⟪———

I ran all the way.

—Harry S. Truman, upon receiving a call on April 12, 1945 to come to the White House

———⟫•⟪———

What makes running an integral part of someone's life? That may be an unanswerable question. Some people have no idea why they wake up every morning and have to get in their run.

—Tom Fleming

I tell runners . . . that no matter how inexperienced a runner you may be, there is nothing wrong with being intense. You don't know what you might discover.
—Francie Larrieu Smith

Running with your dog is probably one of the safest things you can do for yourself, and it can be great for the animal as well.
—Mimi Noonan, DVM

In addition to the safety factor, we run together for companionship, and to remind each other how important a part of our lives this activity is.
—Gordon Bloch

Coaching is no different from what a choreographer does with a dance or what a playwright does with a play.
—Brooks Johnson, Stanford University coach

My philosophy on running is, I don't dwell on it, I do it.
—Joan Samuelson

Everyone needs a good coach. That person is like an outside observer, another set of eyes.
  —Toshiko D'Elia

———✦———

As a coach, I try to keep people from taking their running too seriously.
  —Gordon Bloch

———✦———

I've been running for over 20 years; I read all the books and articles, yet I need a coach. Why? I still have to be told, to be encouraged.
  —Fred Lebow

———✦———

I have a few requirements about who I will coach. I think a person has to stay with a program at least one year. That's the only way to know if it works. If I sense an athlete won't stick with a program, I won't work with him or her.
  —Tom Fleming

———✦———

I'm conscious of every little pain and discomfort, from constipation to a side stitch. I have a new relationship to that pain. I don't fight it anymore; I respect my pain.
  —Fred Lebow

I have even cried once or twice when I crossed the finish line, out of a fullness of feeling that can't be expressed in words.
—Larry Smith

It's been proven that you can run, and run well, at age 40 and beyond. It's not merely a younger person's sport.
—Priscilla Welch

Success does not come to the most righteous and rigorously disciplined but to those who continue running.
—Amby Burfoot

[I]t's only something normal for a sportsman to retire. You cannot control the whole world forever. People soon forget you because another champion comes along.
—Haile Gebrselassie

I'm not doing what society dictates. I have no children. I run for a living.
—Francie Larrieu Smith

If it's fun and sweaty, just go out and do it.
—Amby Burfoot

Sometimes, on days I'm truly not motivated, I use errands to make me run. I carry a plastic bag or small backpack and run to the store to shop.
—Ana Da Silva

Running is my sunshine.
—Joan Twine

[O]n days when I'm not motivated, I reason that I'd rather put in one hour of drudgery to gain 23 hours of bliss. Bliss means that for the rest of the day, I'm not guilty about drinking a beer, watching a football game, taking a nap.
—Stuart Witt

To really keep things light, at times I prefer silly running. I find a friend of similar temperament and we plan what I call bozo runs—like running with jingle bells on during Christmas season or costumes at Halloween.
—Tom Allen

Bill Rodgers probably has more physical talent than anyone I've ever met, but his relaxed attitude under pressure is what distinguishes him.

—Tom Fleming

Some running should be different mentally just the way it is different physically. On my easy runs, I may use the time to relax and let my mind wander, but I never do that in hard workouts or races.

—Grete Waitz

Movement is almost synonymous with life.

—Bernd Heinrich, *Why We Run: A Natural History*

When you run in places you visit, you encounter things you'd never see otherwise.

—Tom Brokaw

At eighteen miles the lead runners began to catch up with me, whizzing by as if I was going backward. Bill Rodgers passed me by, yelling, "Thataboy, Dick." That had to be one of the most exciting thrills of my life.

—Dick Traum, the first amputee to run the New York City Marathon

There were no spectators, only goats. I actually have a special feeling for goats, as we used to have them at home when I was growing up. But they don't make for a great cheering section.

—Fred Lebow on running the Aruba Marathon

I loved cross country right from the start. I loved the open territory and going the distance.

—Bill Rodgers

You're . . . better off having the same attitude in business as you have for successful running.

—Alberto Salazar

He was going to grind the opposition into the earth, and if he ground himself in the process, that was too bad.

—William R. Loader, "Staying the Distance"

Running prowess may seem unimportant to an antelope until that rare moment in its life when a lion gives chase.

—Bernd Heinrich, *Why We Run: A Natural History*

Walking or running makes us part of the living cosmic unity, and that is not something restricted to the young.
　　　　—Roger Robinson

———✦———

One of my biggest desires as a coach is to help adults learn to run like they did as kids. It's such a natural movement when kids do it.
　　　　—T'ai Chi master George Xu

———✦———

In Antarctica you don't just need physical strength. You also need courage and wisdom.
　　　　—William Tan, wheelchair participant in the Antarctica Marathon

———✦———

You can jog while pushing a baby carriage.
　　　　—Nina Kucsik

———✦———

The numbers are in and they show women's running is hot.
　　　　—Gloria Averbuch

Years ago, women sat in kitchens drinking coffee and discussing life. Today, they cover the same topics while they run.

—Joan Benoit Samuelson

The way I see it, you have to view running time not as extra or wasted time, but as important, productive contemplation time.

—Fred Lebow

Gazelles run when they're pregnant. Why should it be any different for women?

—Joan Ullyot, M.D.

Don't automatically head for a high-tech shoe. I think you should only wear as much shoe as you need for your body to work as efficiently as it can.

—Tom Hartge, Nike

Use goals not as ends in themselves but as stepping stones. When you reach 80 percent of your long-range goal, reset it.

—Dr. Linda Bunker, sports psychologist

Success is 90 percent physical and 10 percent mental. But never underestimate the power of that 10 percent.
—Tom Fleming

⇒◆⇐

You don't want your competition to know what's ailing you.
—Dick Beardsley

⇒◆⇐

Ultimately, the best runners are the ones who are willing to work very hard but who have a little bit of a lazy streak in them.
—Benji Durden, coach

⇒◆⇐

Somewhere along the path, running became the canvas upon which I documented my life.
—Dagny Scott, *Runners World Complete Book of Women's Running*

⇒◆⇐

I race in order to dig deep within myself and see what I'm really made of.
—Maggie, runner from Idaho

The surprising part is that women are usually more sensible than men. I find this in their approach to sports in general . . . they seem more willing to listen to so-called voices of authority, or reason.

  —Gordon Bloch

<hr />

Running is not only physical. If it were, you could put a great bull-like guy to it and he'd break every record.

  —Denis Johansson

<hr />

Given the nature of running, certain things will never be altered. That's one of the beauties of our sport. There is no judge; it doesn't matter how you look.

  —Bill Rodgers

<hr />

I don't stop until the world gets gray and fuzzy around the edges.

  —Candi Clark

<hr />

Do they tackle you in cross-country?

  —Dick Beardsley to a friend in high school

Accept your limitation and, with care, the thinking runner will have a comfortable, creditable race. But go for broke and prepare to be broken.
—George Sheehan

———◆———

It turned out that no one without the standard issue of two working legs had ever run a marathon before. It took me seven hours and twenty-four minutes to finish and the excitement generated at that race hasn't stopped yet.
—Dick Traum on running the New York City Marathon in 1976

———◆———

You feel good while you're running and you feel even better when you're finished.
—Fred Lebow

———◆———

Compared to a lot of runners, I'm not very loyal to my running shoes.
—Sarah Bowen Shea

———◆———

Running has always helped keep me sane, so I thought running could help these guys burn off energy and stress.
—Laura Bowman, who is in charge of a running club for prisoners

He lived only for running. He got up in the morning and walked to the school for it, waiting all day for that living half hour when he emerged on the playing field and ran, suffering, until he swore he would never do it again, and at last finished somehow and returned to the locker room.

—James Buechler, "John Sobieski Burns"

Running has given me an opportunity to reach out and be a benefit to a fellow human being.

—Mark Goldstein on the Komen Race for the Cure, a 5K that raises breast cancer awareness

Most runners want to run either longer or faster at some point in their running career, but without good running form, added distance will only lengthen the time you are running improperly and increase your odds of getting hurt.

—George Xu

I'm just doing what I love to do—swimming, biking, running—whether I have legs or not. If I had legs, I might not be as active.

—Rudy Garcia-Tolson, who can run a 5.57-minute mile on two prosthetic legs

Running is the space in my day when I feel the most beautiful—when I don't feel judged by others. And that's what I want for all little girls.
    —Molly Barker, founder of Girls on the Run International

—◆—

My eyes burned with sweat, and I squinted so tight I could hardly see anymore, and because they stung it was impossible to think. I was adjusting, though, lost in rhythm, like a mechanical animal caught on the rim of existence . . . it felt good and I was slipping deep in dreams.
    —Walter McDonald, "The Track"

—◆—

I give my staff my running schedule six months in advance. God help them if they put something on top of it.
    —Former Arkansas Governor Mike Huckabee

—◆—

It is the illusion that we can go no faster that holds us back.
    —Kenny Moore

—◆—

I'm willing to accept any kind of pain to win a race.
    —Rick Wohlhutter

Running gives me confidence.
    —Steve Prefontaine

As athletes—even just by who we are and how we live—we are able to pass on a great gift to other women and girls.
    —Gloria Averbuch

I felt like I could see and hear everything. When I crossed the finish line that afternoon, I felt glorious, like I was going to live forever.
    —David Hobler on the 1982 Boston Marathon

My body immediately reacts to a lack of exercise. "Take me outside," it cries, "let me out."
    —Paula Zahn

I was hurting from sheer physical exhaustion, but when I heard the cheering, it carried me along. I wasn't going to stop now. The last quarter mile, when the crowds were at their peak, they roared as if I was running down a football field for the winning touchdown.
    —Dick Traum, the first amputee to run the New York City Marathon

So much in life seems inflexible and unchangeable, and part of the joy of running and especially racing is the realization that improvement and progress can be achieved.

  —Nancy Anderson

———————

I love running because you feel so good.

  —Barbara Orr

———————

I knew I had disciplined myself, that running was my own doing. I knew that no one had pushed me to do it. I knew that I was able to accomplish what I had because I had worked on it.

  —Nina Kuscik

———————

Life is complicated. Running is simple. Is it any wonder that people like to run?

  —Kevin Nelson, *The Runner's Book of Daily Inspiration*

———————

If you become restless, speed up. If you become winded, slow down. You climb the mountain in a equilibrium between restlessness and exhaustion.

  —Robert Pirsig

I have two doctors: my left leg and my right.
—George M. Trevelyan

———◆———

It is better, I think, to begin easily and get your running to be smooth and relaxed and then to go faster and faster.
—Henry Rono

———◆———

Methinks that the moment my legs began to move, my thoughts began to flow.
—Henry David Thoreau

———◆———

Cross country is like being a mountain goat, picking your way over roots and rocks, leaping over logs. It's grueling; it takes a lot of heart. But the rewards are great.
—Lynn Jennings

———◆———

After a week of the contained chaos that is my job, I need some solitary running time. On Sundays, I can unwind and reconnect with the natural world.
—Linda Jones

It's best to approach your break point without breaking it.

    —Lee Fidler, running coach

———◆———

Running long and hard is an ideal antidepressant, since it's hard to run and feel sorry for yourself at the same time. Also, there are those hours of clearheadedness that follow a long run.

    —Monte Davis

———◆———

We are what we repeatedly do. Excellence, then, is not an act, but a habit.

    —Aristotle

———◆———

There's nothing quite like the feeling you get from knowing you're in good physical condition. I wake up alert and singing in the morning, ready to go.

    —Stan Gerstein

———◆———

The sanity of runners is also called into question, since we can sometimes be found slowly moving up and down the driveway while staring at a watch.

    —Bob Schwartz, *I Run, Therefore I Am—Nuts*

I knew that women were capable of running marathons if they were only given the opportunity.

    —Kathrine Switzer

———⟫◆⟪———

The runner's greatest asset, apart from essential fitness of body, is a cool and calculating brain allied to confidence and courage.

    —Franz Stampfl, *Franz Stampfl on Running*

———⟫◆⟪———

Get out of my race!

    —Boston Marathon official Jock Semple to Kathrine Switzer in 1967

———⟫◆⟪———

Passion is running and running is passion.

    —Gail W. Kislevitz

———⟫◆⟪———

The confident Hare took off at top speed . . . lollopped along, feeling pleased with its own brilliance . . . and stopped for a nap. . . . The determined Tortoise kept patiently padding and plodding along without any pause, until quietly it waddled past the sleeping Hare.

    —Aesop

We don't let any grass grow under our feet, we're too busy running!
—Kim Ahrens

———◦———

I knew if I quit, nobody would ever believe that women had the capability to run the marathon distance.
—Kathrine Switzer

———◦———

That day remains very special to me and if I had one day to live over in my lifetime, it would be my first marathon.
—Dick Traum, the first amputee to run the New York City Marathon

———◦———

Scientific testing on the benefits of vitamin, mineral, and herbal preparations is inconclusive at best. This lack of absolute proof doesn't turn runners away from these products. They work because we use the strongest additive of all—faith.
—Joe Henderson, *Running 101*

———◦———

For every runner who tours the world running marathons, there are thousands who run to hear the leaves and listen to the rain, and look to the day when it is suddenly as easy as a bird in flight.
—George Sheehan

I've been running a lot of open races against Kenyans and they like to blow it out hard in the beginning . . . it's a little scary doing that because you can just die out there doing that.
  —Mike Mykytok

When I run with someone else, the conversation flows naturally because . . . what else can we do?
  —Amby Burfoot, *The Runner's Guide to the Meaning of Life*

Almost thirty years ago, I lined up for my first marathon. Little did I know then how much that event would change my life.
  —Grete Waitz, *Run Your First Marathon*

No, Jackie, this isn't a coach-athlete thing. This is your husband telling you its time for you to go.
  —Bob Kersee, coach to Jackie Joyner-Kersee, asking her to retire

If you train intelligently and have the right gear, you can continue to enjoy the fitness and general sense of well-being that accompanies running while avoiding running injuries.

—*The U.S. Navy Seal Guide to Fitness and Nutrition*

———◆———

These frenzied spectators literally overwhelmed him, swarming round, shouting, yelling, dancing and jumping about like madmen. Those who got near him slapped and banged him on the back, yelling as they did so, "Good!" "Splendid!" "Glorious!" Thus they continued until all the little remaining breath in George's body was well-nigh beaten out of him.

—account from an unnamed newspaper about Walter Goodall
    George's victory in a running event with William Cummings in
    England in 1886

———◆———

Pain is a given. I don't try to fight the pain or pretend it's not there. In fact, I give into it. But only for a little while.

—Ric Munoz

———◆———

The marathon has been referred to as a person's horizontal Everest.

—Grete Waitz and Gloria Averbuch, *Run Your First Marathon*

I'm rapidly getting to the point now where I don't care about the interviews or anything anymore. I guess from a business point of view every bit of publicity you can get is good, but it's just not worth it to me. You get sick about talking about the same thing over and over again.

    —Alberto Salazar

———◆———

It was a lifetime of training for just 10 seconds.

    —Jesse Owens, on the Olympics

———◆———

Don't let anybody kid you. Runners make runners. Coaches like to take all the credit, but day after day, the upper classmen show the younger fellows how to run, how to train, how to take care of themselves.

    —Jumbo Elliot

———◆———

Winning is always satisfying, but when you succeed in a marathon, it stays with you. . .You will feel the sweetness of the achievement forever.

    —Grete Waitz and Gloria Averbuch, *Run Your First Marathon*

Everyone knows about the bear. He's that invisible animal that waits for you about a hundred yards from the finish line. He jumps on your back and starts clawing and scratching and he seems so heavy that you want to stop running so that he'll get off and leave you alone.

  —Bruce Jenner

CHAPTER TWELVE

On the marathon and beyond

Going the Distance

With a half dozen miles to go in a marathon, Frank Shorter commented to friendly rival Kenny Moore, "Too bad Pheidippides didn't die at 20 miles."

But would the magic of the marathon remain if the distance had been anything less than the admittedly quirky 26 miles 385 yards? Would we still see nearly 40,000 runners lined up on starting lines from Chicago to New York to London to Berlin?

Possibly, but if we appeased Frank and lowered the bar, it would remove from the race a significant challenge. Scientists tell us that we can store enough glycogen in our muscles to get us to the 20-mile mark, the so-called "Wall." Those who train using one of my programs get to that distance in their last long run and stop without significantly having tested themselves. Intermediate and Advanced runners following my programs run two or three 20-milers. More experienced marathoners run somewhat more often than that, elite runners going that far week after week after week.

But move into that 21st mile, and the 22nd, and the 23rd, and the ones beyond, and it is like punching the button on the treadmill that elevates the belt. Parts start coming off the machine: your machine!

Yes, Frank. Let's leave the distance alone. In your victory at the Olympic Games in Munich, there remained still a few speedy runners in your wake who might have stayed with you had the distance been a more mortal 20 miles. By 26 miles 385 yards, there remained no doubt who was champion that day.

And as runners today cross the finish line at that magical distance, they continue to join you on the victory stand.

If you want to win something, run 100 meters. If you want to experience something, run a marathon.

    —Emil Zatopek

——◆——

When I run a marathon, I put myself at the center of my life, the center of my universe. For these hours, I move past ideas of food and shelter and sexual fulfillment and other basic drives.

    —George Sheehan

——◆——

He was thinking: There is nothing like the Marathon. Just the figures alone mean something: 26 miles, 385 yards.

    —John L. Parker, Jr., *Once a Runner*

——◆——

Aretha Franklin's "Respect" started playing. In my head, I was singing, "R-E-S-P-E-C-T" and suddenly I got that last nudge through the finish.

    —John-Louis Kronfeld, on breaking through "The Wall" at the
       Marine Corps Marathon

Your goal is to keep an even pace or, even better, to speed up at the end, running so-called negative splits. Most runners do the opposite, with devastating results. Every recent world best in the marathon was set by athletes who ran at an even pace or ran negative splits.

 —Gina Kolata, "Keeping the Gauge off 'E,'" *The New York Times,*
  October 25, 2007

———◆———

Years ago, the picture of people running marathons was these lean, mean Type-A male running machines, but today people running are your neighbors, just regular people. It's a different sport now and we have to cater to these new people, not exclude them.

 —Tracy Sundlun, executive Vice President of Elite Racing, on
  opposing the ban on using headphones in races

———◆———

Runners are no longer content with fitness but are seeking a new awareness of the self in the total experience of running—and more often than not they are culminating that quest by running a marathon.

 —George Sheehan

Every serious marathoner should do Boston, to experience the close to a million spectators, the three generations of families out cheering, the little kids handing you water or orange slices. The whole city really appreciates the runners.

      —Neil Weygandt, who had finished 41 straight Boston marathons as of 2007

⸻ ◆ ⸻

The marathon had always been a hand-me-down kind of event. In general, guys went into the marathon because they weren't fast enough at the shorter distances.

      —Bill Squires on marathons in the 1970s

⸻ ◆ ⸻

If people were possessed by reason, running marathons would not work. But we are not creatures of reason. We are creatures of passion.

      —Noel Carroll

⸻ ◆ ⸻

I used to be a runner myself, quite a useful one too but a bit of a plodder.

      —Allan Sillitoe, *The Loneliness of the Long Distance Runner*

Carbo-loading will only get you twenty miles. For the last six you eat your heart out. In my training, even with Gatorade and bee pollen and seventy-dollar heel inserts, I can't make it past twenty miles.

—Max Apple, "Carbo-Loading"

A miler's kick does the trick. . . . A miler's kick does the trick. . .

—Rod Dixon's mental refrain as he chased down and beat Geoff Smith in the last half mile of the 1983 New York City Marathon

No doubt a brain and some shoes are essential for marathon success, although if it comes down to a choice, pick the shoes. More people finish marathons with no brains than with no shoes.

—Don Kardong

Never stand directly in front of a runner after they've finished a marathon. It's a mistake you make only once—and it'll cost you a pair of shoes.

—John Bingham, "You're in Good Hands," *Runners World*

It is important to keep the marathon in perspective. Running does not have to be the controlling element in your life, but if you become a marathon runner it probably will be, for a while.
　　　—Marc Bloom, *The Runner's Bible*

———◆———

The marathon . . . is, to use Yeats's description of poetry, "blood, imagination, and intellect brought together."
　　　—George Sheehan

———◆———

[I]n an unequal world, in this one endeavor people of vastly differing abilities share something in common: the act of going the distance. Whether it's two hours or four or five, the effort and achievement are similar.
　　　—Fred Lebow

———◆———

What is the great appeal of the marathon? This is something I continually ask myself as nearly 50,000 requests for entries pour in every year for the New York City Marathon.
　　　—Fred Lebow

Running a marathon is a tremendous accomplishment. I never understood why people ran them until I did it. Crossing the finish line of my first marathon gave me that "first-time glow"—a sense of accomplishment that I have not felt since.
—Francie Larrieu Smith

———✦———

The marathon is a bizarre event, and as a coach I hate it.
—Bob Sevene

———✦———

Almost every first-time marathoner says the same thing at the finish line: "Never again."
—Bob Glover, *The Runner's Handbook*

———✦———

I viewed every marathon as a test of my manhood.
—Alberto Salazar

———✦———

Water: It's the most important part of a marathon. And so many times there isn't enough.
—Fred Lebow

Marathon training is no great mystery. Don't throw your current training out the window in search of that "magic" marathon program.
　　—Grete Waitz

[The marathon is] kind of like the Ph.D. of public fitness accomplishments. There are very few times as an adult that you can go out and do something that's authentically difficult and be publicly lauded for it.
　　—Marcy in Cate Terwilliger's "Marathon Woman"

One of the scariest things about running a marathon for the first time isn't the distance, the muscle pain, the chafing, or the blisters. It's not knowing what's going to happen.
　　—*Runner's World UK*

The standard prayer to St. Michael is, "St. Michael the Archangel, defend us on the day of battle, be our protection against the wickedness and snares of the devil." For me, marathon day is a battle and the last six miles are where the devil lays his snares and I ask St. Michael to help me out.
　　—Larry Smith

I've dropped out of many marathons. I'm not proud of it. I feel terrible dropping out, but if I have to do it, I do. It's part of the game, and often gives you the impetus to do better in the future.

  —Fred Lebow

I tend to run better if I put in very high mileage the week *before* I start my four-day countdown.

  —Bill Rodgers on preparing for a marathon

It's a poor man's race. You don't have to go to college or belong to any club, and there's nothing in it but a medal and a cup if you win. And yet they've been running this race for over forty years. There have been marathons ever since the Greeks defeated the Persians.

  —Kay Reynolds in George Harmon Coxe's "See How They Run"

Almost every first-time marathoner says the same thing at the finish line: "Never again."

  —Bob Glover, *The Runner's Handbook*

Those long runs cleanse my system, physically and mentally.
—Joan Benoit Samuelson

It is true that speed kills. In distance running, it kills anyone who does not have it.
—Brooks Johnson

There is the truth about the marathon and very few of you have written the truth. Even if I explain to you, you'll never understand it, you're outside of it.
—Douglas Wakiihuri, speaking to journalists

Baby boomers in general and boomer distance runners in particular were heirs both to the warrior mentality of their World War II-veteran fathers and the new consciousness of the 1960s and '70s. Both ways of thinking were essentially idealistic and challenged us to adopt causes greater than ourselves. The marathon served as an ideal outlet for both types of energy.
—Tom Derderian

I still think the marathon is easy, if you are mentally and physically prepared for it.

    —Steve Jones

———◆———

At mile 80, it's not all that great, but you live through it and then fondly recall how good it was.

    —Tim Twietmeyer, winner of five 100-mile Western States
       Endurance Runs

———◆———

Marathons are extraordinarily difficult, but if you've got the training under your belt, and if you can run smart, the races take care of themselves.

    —Deena Kastor, first American woman to run a marathon under 2:20

———◆———

I definitely want to show how beautiful the marathon can be. I am the opponent of all those who find the marathon bad: the psychologists, the physiologists, the doubters. I make the marathon beautiful for myself and for others. That's why I'm here.

    —Uta Pippig

I have been asked everywhere I go: Why do people run the marathon? Sure, there is a sense of status we gain among our peers. But I think the real reasons are more personal. I think it is because we need to test our physical, emotional, or creative abilities.

—Fred Lebow

———⟫•⟪———

If people were possessed by reason, running marathons would not work. But we are not creatures of reason. We are creatures of passion.

—Noel Carroll

———⟫•⟪———

It is a sublime thing to suffer and be stronger.

—Henry Wadsworth Longfellow

———⟫•⟪———

I felt like I played in a very rough football game with no hitting above the waist.

—Alan Page, former NFL player

———⟫•⟪———

You can actually suffer a little bit more going slowly than when you're going really fast. A faster marathon might even be easier than a slow one, in terms of what it takes out of you mentally.

—Frank Shorter

Even today, twenty-one years later, I still get chills when I remember [the roar of the crowd at the Boston Marathon in 1982]. It echoed and reverberated into this deafening, almost palpable wall of sound. It was very powerful. It sounded almost holy.

—John Lodwick

———◆———

As he staggered, half-blind in the dim light, to the foot of the hill, he thought of the Athenian runner finishing the first Marathon and, as he collapsed, crying, "Rejoice, we conquer!" Nilson realized how much that image, those words had been with him, influencing him all his life. They heartened him now, sealed the sense of meaning in him.

—Harry Sylvester, "Going to Run All Night"

———◆———

At the two-thirds mark, I think of those who are still with me. Who might make a break? Should I? Then I give it all I've got.

—Ibrahim Hussein

———◆———

Being able to run fast means nothing, if you haven't trained your body to throw in a 4:40 mile at mile 25.

—Ryan Lamppa

I'm never going to run this again.
> —Grete Waitz, after winning her first of nine New York City marathons

⟡

The marathon can humble you.
> —Bill Rodgers

⟡

I can't accept this marathon business: who wants to run 26 miles and 385 yards, in a competitive race? Jane does. For the last three months at least our lives have been taken over by those 26 miles, what we eat, what we do, where we go, and I have learned to hate every one of them.
> —Sara Maitland, "The Loveliness of the Long-Distance Runner"

⟡

When I knew I was going to win in 2004, I still felt awful. The last mile, I was just managing how much I was going to die.
> —Alan Culpepper, winner of the 2004 U.S. Olympic Marathon Trials

⟡

I am too tired even to be happy.
> —Gelindo Bordin, after winning the marathon at the Helsinki Olympics

The Boston Marathon has had more to do with liberating and promoting women's marathoning than any other race in the world.
  —Joe Henderson

For most runners, the marathon is like rolling dice.
  —Bob Sevene

Get going. Get up and walk if you have to, but finish the damned race.
  —Ron Hill to Jerome Drayton during the 1970 Boston Marathon

---

The New York Marathon: a fantastic event.
  —Pope John Paul II, 1982

The starting line of the New York City marathon is kind of a giant time bomb behind you about to go off.
  —Bill Rodgers

Running cross-country is the closest man will ever get to flying.
 —Joseph VanderStel

The freedom of cross-country is so primitive. It's woman versus nature.
 —Lynn Jennings

I was running to catch a train when one of my teachers saw me. He thought I was fast, timed me, and later gave me my first instructions in sprinting. I happened to be in the right place at the right time.
 —Elizabeth Robinson Schwartz

The marathon is the focal point of all that has gone before and all that will come afterward.
 —George Sheehan

Road racing is rock 'n roll; track is Carnegie Hall.
 —Marty Liquori

If you are going to do a marathon, decide what drink you are going to use way ahead of time, and use it in your long training runs.

    —Priscilla Welch on energy drinks

<hr>

[T]he Médoc Marathon serves wine at its water stops. First prize is the winner's weight in grand crus.

    —Benjamin Cheever, *Strides*

<hr>

Any idiot can run a marathon. It takes a special kind of idiot to run an ultramarathon.

    —Alan Cabelly

<hr>

Training to run 100 miles is like training to get hit by a truck.

    —Luis Escobar

<hr>

If you feel good while running the Western States 100-mile Endurance Run, don't worry. You'll get over it.

    Gene Thibeault

The race continued as I hammered up the trail, passing rocks and trees as if they were standing still.
　　—Red Fisher, on his Wasatch Front 100 in 1986

—◆—

Surprisingly, the "idea" of running a hundred miles didn't frighten me. Instead, it awakened in me a curiosity, a wonder in myself, my ability, my strength, both physical and mental, and a quiet want. . . . I simply let it live inside me for a while, months, a year, two years, until I felt it coming out as stronger than just a murmur.
　　—Kris Whorton

—◆—

If God invented marathons to keep people from doing anything more stupid, the triathlon must have taken Him completely by surprise.
　　—P. Z. Pearce

—◆—

The first fifty miles are run with the legs, the second fifty with the mind.
　　—Anonymous

—◆—

If you have a weak spot, the marathon will let you know.
　　—Frank Shorter

When you run there are no mistakes, only lessons. The art and science of ultra-running is a process of trial, error and experimentation. The failed experiments are as much a part of the process as the combination that ultimately works.

—Keith Pippin

—————

I really like cross-country. You're one with the mud.

—Lynn Jennings

—————

I often leave my trusty routes through the country woods to explore new areas. Where does that road lead to? What is at the top of that hill?

—Bob Glover, *The Runner's Handbook*

—————

The marathon is charismatic. It has everything. It has drama. It has competition. It has camaraderie. It has heroism.

—Fred Lebow

—————

Run too far and the body doesn't want to stop.

—Richard Christian Matheson, "Third Wind"

The marathon is my benchmark. It is the status symbol in my community, the running community.

  —George Sheehan

       —◆—

I am not entirely happy about the popularity of the marathon. Too many runners feel an obligation to run it. It is as though they cannot feel they are serious runners until they have met the challenge of the marathon.

  —Marc Bloom, *The Runner's Bible*

       —◆—

There's a park across the street from the house where I grew up. It took me a while to work up to running "all the way around the park." When I finally did, it was a really big deal. I ran all the way around the park! "You did what? All the way around? My goodness!" Everyone in my family was impressed. I had to lie down for the rest of the day. I measured it later—nine-tenths of a mile.

  —Tish Hamilton, executive editor at *Runner's World*

       —◆—

I like hills because you can see the top. I know that sounds glib, but you know that the hill is not going to keep appearing; it's there and once you get to the top, it's behind you, and you feel as though you have conquered something.

  —Rob de Castella

In an ultra you should eat like a horse, drink like a fish, and run like a turtle.
—Anonymous

◆

I was out training one black night when I heard a noise. I turned around and saw a leopard. I threw some stones at him and he went away, so I went on my way.
—Filbert Bayi on running in his native Tanzania

◆

Running cross country is the closest man will ever get to flying.
—Joseph VanderStel

◆

All men may not be brothers, but that's the way it feels after a marathon. . . . You feel—you can't help but feel—that you all understand each other.
—Benjamin Cheever, *Strides*

◆

The greatest treadmill running song, of course, is "Black Dog" from *Led Zeppelin IV*.
—Pete Pfitzinger

I never met a hill I couldn't walk.
>   —Larry Stice

—◆—

Most often . . . the women who saw me looked stunned; they didn't know how to react. . . . I wanted to say, "Yes, it's eighteen miles and I've run that far, and I will go twenty-six. Women *can* do this."
>   —Kathrine Switzer on running marathons

—◆—

My introduction to track racing was through the background of cross country running, which is not a sport perhaps as popular in America as it is in England.
>   —Roger Bannister

—◆—

My dad was working out on the treadmill when Governor Bush called and officially asked him to be his running mate.
>   —Mary Cheney

—◆—

I love running cross country . . . on a track, I feel like a hamster.
>   —Robin Williams

I've always liked hills. I see a challenge, a goal, and I feel instantly galvanized to achieve the goal.

—Amby Burfoot, *The Runner's Guide to the Meaning of Life*

———⊰◦⊱———

A marathon is like life with its ups and downs, but once you've done it you feel that you can do anything.

—Anonymous

———⊰◦⊱———

When you run a marathon, you mean it. We're built for running. We dream of flying. For now, though, we're built to run.

—Benjamin Cheever, *Strides*

———⊰◦⊱———

To describe the agony of a marathon to someone who's never run it is like trying to explain color to someone who was born blind.

—Jerome Drayton

———⊰◦⊱———

Marathon running is a terrible experience: monotonous, heavy, and exhausting.

—Veikko Karvonen, 1954 Europe and Boston Marathon champion

You have to forget your last marathon before you try another. Your mind can't know what's coming.

—Anonymous

⎯⎯◆⎯⎯

I did philosophy from miles five to eleven, trying to form one discriminating sentence about Socrates, Kant, Spinoza, Kierkegaard, whomever. When I came to the authors of *How to Be Your Own Best Friend*, I knew my mind was wandering and let go of systematizing.

—Max Apple, "Carbo-Loading"

⎯⎯◆⎯⎯

I once ran thirty-one miles and after that there was nothing in the world I thought I couldn't do.

—Kathrine Switzer

⎯⎯◆⎯⎯

There is reason for viewing with considerable apprehension the sudden popularity of the so-called Marathon race. . . . It is only exceptional men who can safely undertake the running of twenty-six miles, and even for them the safety is comparative rather than absolute.

—*The New York Times*, February 24, 1909

The long race is there always, as a sort of platform on which to evaluate, and sometimes alter your life.
    —Benjamin Cheever, *Strides*

———✦———

The natural urge when running a distance is to push harder and finish sooner—to race against time. Every second behind a deadline is a little defeat.
    —Joe Henderson

———✦———

[The marathon is] kind of like the Ph.D. of public fitness accomplishments. There are very few times as an adult that you can go out and do something that's authentically difficult and be publicly lauded for it.
    —Marcy in Cate Terwilliger's "Marathon Woman"

———✦———

When I'm training for a marathon, I soak in a hot tub every day, and get a weekly masssage.
    —Anne Marie Lauck

———✦———

And this long-distance running lark is the best of all, because it makes me think so good that I learn things even better than when I'm on my bed at night.
    —Alan Sillitoe in "The Loneliness of Long-Distance Running"

The marathon is the ultimate endurance test. Oh, sure, some people sometimes go longer than that. But 26 miles 385 yards is where racing ends and where ludicrous extremes begin.

—Joe Henderson

———◆———

The winners run at speeds equaled or surpassed by no more than a handful of runners ever in the world. As important for me was the fact that more than fifteen thousand people from sixty-eight countries compete in our race.

—Fred Lebow, organizer of the New York City Marathon

———◆———

To understand the marathon is to run it a lot. . . . You can't really know it until you've felt the other side of it. That's the only way it's possible.

—Bill Rodgers

———◆———

To the spectators, it's a freak show with legs; to the legitimate runners, it's a test of speed and endurance; and to the exhibitionists, it's a chance to be a screwball before a ready-made gallery.

—Will Cloney

[Y]ou have to respect the distance, which is often said about marathons but applies equally to all distance running.

    —Amby Burfoot, *The Runner's Guide to the Meaning of Life*

———◆———

After every experience, it's natural to reflect that you might have done better. Only after a marathon can I say I have given everything.

    —Kenny Moore

———◆———

I wanted to try a marathon.

    —Grete Waitz, when asked why she had come to her fist New York City Marathon

CHAPTER THIRTEEN

Long may you run

Finish Line

Each morning when we are at our winter home in Ponte Vedra Beach, Florida, I purchase the local newspaper, which includes a schedule of tides—high and low. I check this schedule daily. My life revolves around it. I run each day at low tide.

Low tide is when the beach is widest and flattest, thus, best for running. At high tide, the beach all but vanishes. Only a tiny slab of shore remains between ocean and houses. It is slanted, loose, often encrusted with shells and difficult for running.

Each day brings two low tides and two high tides, but not always at the same times. Low tide shifts forward approximately an hour each day, moving from morning to noon to afternoon to evening over a period of time. Thus, to know the best times to run, checking the schedule becomes essential.

As a committed, lifetime runner, I always have enjoyed running in scenic areas: through the woods, in the mountains, along the beach. But as that runner, I often ran past the scenery too fast to see it. Now as I have aged, I also have slowed. This low tide in my life finally has allowed me to slow down and, in effect, sniff the flowers.

Illness or injuries sometimes force runners into low tides, when we must modify activities to recover for high tides to come. Philosophers and physiologists might even argue over whether low and high tides represent low and high points in our lives. They could be either or both. They might be the opposite. More important, they represent change.

As a runner whose fastest days have passed, I may be at the point of low tide in my life. But it remains a very good time to run.

I've covered myriad teams where the fourth quarterback or third-string point guard is barely a part of things; where other players look down on him as

inferior. There is a communal bond among harriers that I've yet to discover in another sport. Doing it *is* good enough in running. . .
　　—Jeff Pearlman, "Heady Days: How a Lousy Collegiate Runner
　　　　Eventually Made It to the Top"

———◆———

Running has never failed to give me great end results, and that's why I keep coming back for more!
　　—Sasha Azevedo

———◆———

Running is a big question mark that's there each and every day. It asks you, "Are you going to be a wimp or are you going to be strong today?"
　　—Peter Maher

———◆———

I never thought I'd have such a luxurious life. A healthy husband . . . beautiful little girl . . . Jacuzzi and beer and fruit bowl and Beethoven and Mendelssohn and running . . . Running is the best thing.
　　—Miki Gorman

[T]he effects of running are not extraordinary at all . . . It is the other states . . . that are peculiar, for they are an abnegation of the way you and I are supposed to feel. As runners, I think we reach directly back along the endless chain of history.

   —James W. Fixx, *The Complete Book of Running*

Life is short. Running makes it seem longer.

   —Baron Hansen

We run because it makes us feel like winners, no matter how slow or how fast we go.

   —Florence Griffith Joyner and John Hanc, *Running for Dummies*

My feeling is that any day I am too busy to run is a day that I am too busy.

   —John Bryant

I am already preparing for the day when I can't run at the top. Maybe I'll do more business, or just become a jogger.

   —Haile Gebrselassie

The woods are lovely dark and deep.
But I have promises to keep,
And miles to go before I sleep,
And miles to go before I sleep.
—Robert Frost, "Stopping by Woods on a Snowy Evening"

Great is the victory, but the friendship of all is greater.
—Emil Zatopek

It should make us proud to know we are part of a running lineage that stretches back from the original Olympic Games in 776 BC to this very moment.
—Michael Sandrock

As I have aged, my running times and goals have changed, and so have my inspirations. I used to idolize the Olympic greats—the Paavo Nurmis, the Emil Zatopeks, the Abebe Bikilas, the Frank Shorters. Now I have a different hero—"Old John" Kelley, who has run the Boston Marathon sixty times.
—Amby Burfoot

Vary your training, your running partners, and your environment. Only your imagination limits the ways you can spice up your running routine.

—Bob Glover, *The Runner's Handbook*

⟫◆⟪

The secret shared by women runners: running is not just physical exercise but a spiritual, mental, and emotional journey.

—*Runner's Gazette*

⟫◆⟪

Don't worry, everyone slows over time and I recall running slower at forty-three than at forty.

—Bill Rodgers

⟫◆⟪

Just like I hope to be a mother the rest of my life, I hope to be a runner the rest of my life.

—Joan Benoit Samuelson

⟫◆⟪

I plan to be running as long as I can and have no plans to stop.

—Frank Shorter

As he swept forward in line with the others a controlled jubilation came over him. Christ, I'm full of running! he thought. I'm absolutely full of running.
  —Victor Price, "The Other Kingdom"

As we run, we become.
  —Amby Burfoot, *The Runner's Guide to the Meaning of Life*

The true runner is a very fortunate person. He has found something in him that is just perfect.
  —George Sheehan

Tears streamed down my face as I crossed the finish line. I was a new person, a runner.
  —Thomas King

Stay hungry and excited about what you are doing. It won't be forever and ever, because there will be a time when you want to bail out, because you want to do other things.
  —Priscilla Welch

As every runner knows, running is about more than just putting one foot in front of the other; it is about our lifestyle and who we are.

> —Joan Benoit Samuelson

———◆———

I've had my fair share of being dismissed. But I'm only about to turn thirty. And when I finish running, I'm going to be a dangerous woman.

> —Cathy Freeman

———◆———

The old man asked me what I was running from. I was in full stride so I couldn't slow down to answer him. I could only hope that the wind carried my correction of "running toward" to his ears.

> —Nancy LaMar Rodgers

———◆———

[E]ven when I'm eighty, I want to be one of the top three eighty-year-olds at the local races.

> —Steve Stovall

———◆———

Running has gone beyond fitness. The jogging movement, which began as a pursuit of health, has become an experiential quest.

> —George Sheehan

You should not be flying down the home straight. Most of your efforts should have been put forth earlier.
—John Treacy

In my mind, I'm still young. When I go to the starting line, I still perceive myself as racing in the open division.
—Francie Larrieu Smith

My final and favorite ritual is the one I perform when I finish [a marathon]. As soon as I get home I take a long hot bath and drink cold beer in the tub. Then I lie on the bed and drink more beer, eat pretzels, and watch a videotape of the race.
—Larry Smith

Time doesn't stand still, and you don't stand still. Things change within your-self, within your life, and within your sport.
—Priscilla Welch

Wisely and slow. They stumble that run fast.
—Shakespeare, *Romeo and Juliet*

I've run a lot of miles over the years, some fast and some not so fast.
  —Alberto Salazar

Love yourself, for who and what you are; protect your dream and develop your talent to the fullest extent.
  —Joan Benoit Samuelson

Last is just the slowest winner.
  —C. Hunter Boyd

Once you are a runner, it's always there in the back of your head.
  —Bill Rodgers

The more I run, the more I want to run, and the more I live a life conditioned and influenced and fashioned by my running. And the more I run, the more certain I am that I am heading for my real goal: to become the person I am.
  —George Sheehan

It's about time to stop; though don't think I'm not still running, because I am, one way or another.

—Alan Sillitoe, "The Loneliness of the Long-Distance Runner"

———

Pray be always in motion.

—Philip Dormer Stanhope Chesterfield

———

In the longest run of all, your life, you're going to be a winner.

—Amby Burfoot, *The Principles of Running*

———

Keeping my eye on today is about all I'm capable of. And today, I think I'll go for a run.

—John Bingham, "Back to the Future," *Runners World*

———

A comedian once claimed that all running does is to allow you to die in good health. Okay, I'll buy that.

—Hal Higdon

Remember that if you don't go to the starting line, you will never view the whole course with all its possibilities. And you will certainly never see the glories of the finish line.

 —Amby Burfoot, *The Runner's Guide to the Meaning of Life*

Often, the enjoyment is the training before and the memory after.

 —Doug Kurtis

If I am still standing at the end of the race, hit me with a board and knock me down, because that means I didn't run hard enough.

 —Steve Jones

Winning has nothing to do with racing. Most days don't have races anyway. Winning is about struggle and effort and optimism, and never, ever, ever giving up.

 —Amby Burfoot, *The Runner's Guide to the Meaning of Life*

These records are only borrowed, precious aspects of the sport, temporarily in one's keeping.

 —Sebastian Coe

You finished a marathon and you believe, "If I can do this, I can do anything."
　　　—Grete Waitz and Gloria Averbuch, *Run Your First Marathon*

—◆—

We walked through the parking lot. Neither of us said anything. We thought the world had ended.
　　　—Anne Ryun, on husband Jim Ryun's retirement

—◆—

Too many runners attempt the marathon much too early in their careers and then become ex-runners.
　　　—Robert Eshich

—◆—

I try to think of myself as an apple tree. Time is not linear, it moves in circles. Come spring, I will bloom again.
　　　—Amby Burfoot, *The Runner's Guide to the Meaning of Life*

—◆—

Sometimes I wonder whether I run high mileage so I can eat like this, or do I eat like this so I can run high mileage?
　　　—Bill Rodgers, on his favorite snack of mayonnaise and chocolate
　　　chip cookies

Rejoice. We conquer!

> —attributed to the Athenian runner who ran from Marathon all the way to Athens to announce the Greek victory over the Persians, and then died.

THOSE QUOTED